ALEXANDER
TECHNIQUE

ALEXANDER TECHNIQUE

ORIGINAL WRITINGS OF
F.M. ALEXANDER

— CONSTRUCTIVE CONSCIOUS CONTROL —

Abridged and edited by
DANIEL MCGOWAN

PUBLISHED FOR THE PAUL BRUNTON
PHILOSOPHIC FOUNDATION BY
LARSON PUBLICATIONS

International Standard Book Number: 0-943914-78-7

Library of Congress Catalog Card Number: 96-76393

Published for the Paul Brunton Philosophic Foundation by
Larson Publications
4936 NYS Route 414
Burdett, NY 14818 USA

03 02 01 00 99 98 97

10 9 8 7 6 5 4 3 2 1

CONTENTS

ACKNOWLEDGEMENTS

Deepest gratitude to Paul and Amy Cash, Anke Dau, Gunda Fielden, Thomas Gwiasda, Sarah Paice and, Gerda and Thoms Törring for their contribution to the production of this text.

FOREWORD

It is now more than a hundred years since Frederick Matthias Alexander (1869–1955) began, as a young man in his twenties, to teach his technique of constructive conscious control of the individual *by the individual*. Nowadays, the Alexander Technique is known to a great number of people around the world from San Francisco to Christchurch. It is taught and practiced in many European countries, in the U.S.A., Australia, New Zealand, Mexico, Brazil, Japan, South Africa, and Israel.

What did Alexander discover? He found the modern human being's use of the self—use of the psycho-physical organism as he called it—which is the universal constant in living, to be in an ever-worsening process of decline. This misuse of the self, he claimed, is the biggest cause of all kinds of neuroses, fears, phobias, and so-called physical ills which plague the modern world. He claimed that the first thing to consider when attempting to alleviate many kinds of illness, is the person's use of the psycho-physical organism in its interaction with people and things in the environment. If someone suffers from misuse of the self, and most of us do, then the person can be taught how to improve it and so to achieve better health.

That a person is taught the Alexander Technique, and not "cured" by it, is an important distinction for the reader to note. This technique is not a therapy, but a process of re-education that almost anyone can learn. Its therapeutic effects, however, can be

tremendous, as Alexander deftly and ably demonstrated throughout his sixty years of teaching it to the public, many of whom came
to him as a last resort when all else had failed.

Alexander himself only discovered this technique as a process of
re-education during his attempts at curing his own throat trouble,
which threatened to cut short his career as an actor and particularly to disrupt his one-man recitations of Shakespeare, his great
love. When he realized that his doctors could not cure his throat
condition, he reasoned that whatever was wrong must be caused
by something he was doing to himself. He then embarked on an
investigation of himself which lasted some nine or ten years,
and which entailed minute observation of his own use with the
help of mirrors.

His investigations led him to realize that his voicework involved
the use of his whole body, which he discovered to be a complex
network of tension patterns from head to toe. Furthermore, he was
startled to see that the mirrors told him he was not doing with his
body what his other sensory feedback was telling him. In other
words, as he later observed to be the case with the vast majority of
us, his "sensory appreciation" had become unreliable.

Traditionally, sensory appreciation is thought of as the instant
fusion by the mind of the information passed to it by the five
senses—hearing, touch, taste, smell, and sight. This instant fusion
forms a perception. There exists, however, a sixth sense which
could be said to have been "lost" or "blocked out." In other words,
a sense of which most of us are only vaguely aware. This sixth sense
is an activity of the nervous system in which sensory nerves connect muscles, tendons, joints, and the middle ear to the brain and
spinal cord. Information travels back and forth telling us, not only
about the interaction of one part of the body with another, but also
of the body's interaction with the environment. This constitutes
our feeling of movement, position, and effort. Current technical
terms for this sense are kinesthesia and proprioception, the two
terms often being used interchangeably.

This sixth aspect of our sensory appreciation plays a highly significant part in determining an individual's perception of stimuli and in determining how he or she will respond to these stimuli. When there is faulty sensory appreciation, every stimulus which comes to a person brings a reaction which registers in the senses (to a greater or lesser degree, according to the level of unreliability) quite differently from that which has actually occurred. Because of individual differences, the same so-called objective stimulus can give different experiences and cause varying emotions, movements, or opinions.

Another important observation that Alexander made was that the co-ordination of the whole mind-body complex depends on the co-ordinated relationship between the head, the neck, and the torso. Through improving the balance of this relationship, his own throat trouble—a specific symptom—disappeared *in the process* of re-educating his use of himself in general. In other words, he found that specific cures for specific illnesses can have only palliative effects and can cause further specific defects in other parts of the organism. He saw that the human being must be re-educated as a whole and not treated specifically. This is still, in these stressful modern times, the blind spot of the society we live in.

Having realized all this, Alexander then went on to make his most important discovery, the process he called *inhibition*— the ability to stop, to stop at the source, those harmful habits of thinking and doing from which most of us suffer. Inhibition in Alexander's sense is a vital function of the nervous system which, when brought up to the conscious level, can enable us to achieve the real psycho-physical-emotional change which so many of us wish for and struggle to attain in our efforts at self-improvement in all spheres of life. Inhibition, so conceived, has nothing to do with suppression. It teaches us how to deal with our stereotyped reactions to the stimuli of living, how to react with reason and poise to those stimuli which we habitually allow to put us wrong.

Alexander realized that the proper place for his technique lay in education, and his main concern was for the person he called his most important client—the child. He founded a school staffed by teachers who also taught his technique and could show the children how to keep, as the first priority, their psycho-physical equilibrium. The children were taught not to be concerned about making mistakes, not to be afraid of failure.

It is important to point out that qualified personal "hands on" instruction is essential in acquiring this technique. As Alexander himself writes, "This whole book is devoted to exposing the fallacy of asking any imperfectly co-ordinated person to attempt to eradicate his or her defects by some written or spoken instructions." Readers are encouraged to contact qualified teachers for a demonstration of this method rather than attempting to practice it without such a demonstration.

During his lifetime, Alexander wrote four books: *Man's Supreme Inheritance, Constructive Conscious Control, The Use of the Self,* and *The Universal Constant in Living.* The four titles run together to give the basis of his teaching as follows: Humanity's supreme inheritance is constructive conscious control in the use of the self which is the universal constant in living. He explains in the books how we can pass from being the slaves of our subconscious, instinctive, and habitual behaviour to conscious, reasoned behaviour and so claim what he called "the transcendent inheritance of a conscious mind."

In reading this abridged, edited version of *Constructive Conscious Control,* the reader is asked to be aware that my aim has been to convey, as accurately as possible, the essential meaning of what Alexander wrote in the original text. I have, therefore, endeavoured to keep the editing of the original text to a minimum, but have made two distinct changes in Alexander's expressions. The first relates to what he called "orders" to denote the passing-on of messages from the mind to the body. The term in popular usage nowadays is "directions" and I have substituted this term for the original "orders." An example of a direction is to "think of not stiffening your neck."

The second change affects his term "means-whereby," which he used in describing the conscious, co-ordinated manner of carrying out any act. I have simply dropped "whereby" and used only the "means."

Any person who has sufficient knowledge and experience of Alexander's work is welcome to send me helpful comments and constructive criticism. I am indebted to Gunda Fielden for her special contribution to the production of this work.

I am the director of a training course for teachers of the Alexander Technique and can be contacted at the following addresses:

> Ausbildungszentrum Für F.M. Alexander Technik
> Borstellstrasse 42
> 12167 Berlin
> Germany

Or

> 11 Bridge Road
> Totnes
> Devon TQ9 5BH
> Great Britain

DANIEL MCGOWAN
APRIL 1996

Constructive Conscious Control of the Individual

F.M. Alexander

PREFACE

The demand for this book has been an insistent one for some time past, particularly from the American readers of *Man's Supreme Inheritance*. Out of gratitude, I have a keen desire to make a contribution to our knowledge worthy of the written encouragement I have received from a large circle of readers, from the Press, and from scientists in Australia, England and America.

I value this mass of correspondence in which requests for further enlightenment are contained. Although it is impossible to answer all of them in this book, I shall give practical illustrations to show, in a general way, the fundamental principles of my methods in the hope that they will help people to a better understanding of the practical side of their problems. I could, indeed, write several volumes and in making my selections for this book I have been influenced by the relative importance of this matter to each portion of my subject. It may, therefore, satisfy disappointed readers to know that I have given due consideration to this essential part of my work.

In *Man's Supreme Inheritance,* I set down my thesis together with practical procedures. Judging from the correspondence received from readers, a better understanding of the *means* to living sanely in the environment of twentieth-century experiences and rapid changes is desired. In this book, I am anxious to answer such questions as: "Why are our instincts less reliable than those of our early ancestors?" "At what stage of humankind's evolution did this deterioration begin?" "What is the cause of our present-day

individual and national unrest?" "Can you give principles which
will enable us to decide what is the best method of educating
our children?" "Evidently your conception of conscious control,
co-ordination, and re-education differs from the usual, so will you
explain this in your next book?" I believe that if I succeed in answering these questions, I shall have made a distinct step forward
in helping to clear away the doubts of any person who is seeking
honestly for truth amidst the mass of methods, systems, "cures,"
and treatments in what are called "physical," "mental," and "spiritual" spheres. It is important to note that enthusiasts for these
different methods point to excellent *specific* results in support of
their contentions; but, in spite of these results, during the past five
hundred years the standard of sensory appreciation, of general co-
ordination and of reliable use of the mechanisms of the organism
has been, and still is, gradually deteriorating.

I will deal with a wide range of more or less generally accepted
statements and principles laid down by experts in these spheres,
so that my readers may decide reliably which system may prove
satisfactory.

To a certain point, I am in sympathy with all workers in either
"physical," "mental," or "spiritual" spheres, because I believe that
"there are more things in heaven and earth than are dreamt of in
our philosophy." But I think that humanity's first duty is to understand and develop those potentialities that are well within the
sphere of our activities here on earth. For this reason I will continue to give practical illustrations to support my arguments. This
formula will, I predict, become more and more the rule, rather
than the exception, because it forces the philosopher to give the
world practical procedures which can be applied to the actual activities of life, instead of theoretical conclusions too often lacking
practical bearing on life. Also, and this is all-important, it transfers
his work from the doubtful field of individual or collective opinion
to the more reliable field of demonstrable conclusion. The philosopher is duty bound to devote years of labor and investigation to the
valuable but difficult process of converting to practical use, every

original idea (opinion). This is a process of years; but if at the end of each experiment, he gives to the world only those ideas which he has succeeded in reducing to practical procedures, rejecting all others, he will make a great contribution to humanity. Philosophy has for centuries too often offered little but personal opinion.

The subject matter of *Man's Supreme Inheritance* shows the need to recognize the unity of human potentialities, instead of seeking solutions to our problems in theories which tend, in practical application, towards separation.

This reference to my thesis allows me to tell readers of the difficulty I have encountered in my attempts to set down, in a sufficiently clear and direct way, the results of my experiences in unfamiliar fields. This difficulty lies in the fact that the adequate description of these experiences, for the purposes of practical application, calls for new and more comprehensive words than we now have at our command. The most appropriate word chosen to convey an idea, will prove inadequate to express the aggregate, after a new element has been added to the idea. In such a case, we are forced either to use an inadequate word or to coin a new one in an attempt to express adequately the expanded idea.

Expanding ideas are the forerunners of human advancement. And the communication of the knowledge concerned with these expanding ideas demands the recognition that new words are needed to express adequately the original as well as the new thought or thoughts involved.

In *Constructive Conscious Control,* the second volume of *Man's Supreme Inheritance,* I am offering constructive arguments and a constructive plan. The fact that I have indulged freely in destructive criticism does not affect this statement, because the aims of this book make this necessary. My criticisms are directed solely towards what I believe to be the impeding factors in our progress towards a constructive plan of life and education.

The preparation of the subject matter of this book has proved a very difficult task, in which I needed considerable assistance. I take this opportunity to express my gratitude to Professor John Dewey for the invaluable suggestions he made after reading the manuscript; to my assistants Ethel Webb and Irene Tasker for their valuable help in and untiring devotion to the work of revising and preparing the subject matter for publication; to Dr. Peter MacDonald and Rev. W.G. Pennyman for assisting me by reading the manuscript and offering criticism; to Mary Olcott for undertaking the responsibility for correction of the proofs; to Edith Lawson and Carla Atkinson for their help with proofs and typescripts. To each and all of these I owe a deep debt of gratitude.

F. MATTHIAS ALEXANDER
16 Ashley Place
Westminster
London, 1923

INTRODUCTION

The principles and procedures of F.M. Alexander are crucially needed at present. Strangely, this is the very reason why they are hard to understand and accept. For although there is nothing esoteric in his teaching and although his exposition is made in simplest English, free from technical words, it is difficult for any- one to grasp its full force without having actual demonstration of the principle in operation. And even then, as I know from personal experience, its full meaning dawns upon one only slowly and with new meanings continually opening up. Since I can add nothing to the clear and full exposition he has given, I think it would be most useful for this introduction to attempt to explain where the difficulty lies in grasping his principle.

The main difficulty, as I have said, lies in the fact that it is so badly needed. The seeming contradiction in this statement is just one instance of the vicious circle which is frequently pointed out and fully dealt with in the text. The principle is badly needed, because in all matters that concern the individual self and the conduct of its life there is a defective and lowered sensory apprecia- tion and judgment, both of ourselves and of our acts, which accompanies our wrongly adjusted psycho-physical mechanisms. It is precisely this perverted consciousness which we bring with us to the reading and comprehension of Alexander's pages and which makes it hard for us to realize his statements as to its existence, causes, and effects. We have become so used to it that we take it for granted. It forms, as he has so clearly shown, our standard of rightness. It influences our every observation, interpretation, and judgment. It is the one factor which enters into our every act and thought.

Consequently, only when the results of F.M. Alexander's lessons have changed one's sensory appreciation and supplied a new standard, so that the old and new conditions can be compared with each other, does the concrete force of his teaching come home to one. In spite of the whole tenor of his teaching, it is this which makes it practically impossible for anyone to go to him with any other idea at the beginning beyond that of gaining some specific relief and remedy. Even after a considerable degree of experience with his lessons, it is possible for one to value his method merely on account of specific benefits received, even though one recognizes that these benefits include a changed emotional condition and a different outlook on life. Only when a pupil reaches the point of giving full attention to F.M. Alexander's *method,* instead of its results, does he realize the constant influence of his sensory appreciation.

The perversion of our sensory consciousness of ourselves has gone so far back that we lack criteria for judging the doctrines and methods that profess to deal with the individual human being. We oscillate between reliance upon plausible general theories and reliance upon testimonies to specific benefits obtained. We oscillate between extreme credulity and complete scepticism. On the one hand, there is the readiest acceptance of all claims of panaceas when these are accompanied by testimonies of personal benefits and cures. On the other hand, the public has seen so many of these panaceas come and go that it has, quite properly, become sceptical about the reality of any new and different principle for developing human well-being.

The world is flooded at present with various systems for relieving ills, such as systems of posture-rectifying exercises, methods of mental, psychological, and spiritual healing, so that, except when an emotional wave is sweeping the country, the very suggestion that there is fundamental truth in an unfamiliar principle is likely to call out the feeling that yet another person has fallen for another one of the "cure-alls" that abound. "How is Alexander's teaching different?" "What assurance is there that it is anything more than these other systems, good for one person, but not another?" If, in reply, specific beneficial results of Alexander's teaching are pointed out, one is reminded that imposing testimonials of this kind can be produced in favor of all the other systems. The point, then, to be decided is: What is the worth of these results and how is their worth to be judged? Or, again, if it is a question of the theories behind the results most of the systems are elaborately reasoned out and claim scientific or spiritual backing. In what fundamental respect do principles and consequences of Alexander's teachings differ from these?

These are fair questions, and it seems to me that probably the best thing to do is to suggest some criteria by which any plan can be judged. Certain other questions may suggest how these criteria may be found. Is a system primarily remedial, curative, aiming at relief of sufferings that already exist, or is it fundamentally preventive in nature? And if preventive rather than corrective, is it specific or general in scope? Does it deal with the "mind" and the "body" as things separated from each other, or does it deal with the unity of the human individuality? Does it aim at securing results directly, by treatment of symptoms, or does it deal with the *causes* of malconditions in such a way that any beneficial results secured come as a natural consequence, almost as by-products of a fundamental change in such conditioning causes? Is it educational in character? If the principle underlying it claims to be preventive and constructive, does it operate from the outside by setting up some automatic safety-device, or does it operate from within? Is it cheap and easy, or does it make demands on the intellectual and moral energies of the individual? Unless it does the latter, what is it but a scheme depending ultimately upon some trick or magic, which, in curing one trouble, is sure to leave behind other troubles (including fixations, inhibitions, lessening of power of steady and intelligent control) since it does not deal with causes, but only directs their operation into different channels and changes perceptible symptoms into more subtle invisible ones?

Bearing such questions in mind when reading Alexander's book allows one to discriminate between the principles of his educational method and those of the systems with which it might be compared and confused.

Any sound plan must prove its soundness both in concrete consequences and in general principles. We too often forget that these principles and facts must not be judged separately, but in connection with each other. Any theory must ultimately be judged by its consequences in operation, and it must be verified experimentally by observation of how it works. In order to justify a claim to be scientific, it must also provide a method for making evident and observable what the consequences are; and this method must afford a guarantee that the observed consequences flow from the principle. And I unhesitatingly assert that, when judged by this standard, Alexander's teaching is scientific in the strictest sense of the word. In other words, Alexander's plan satisfies the most exacting demands of scientific method.

Alexander's theory and the observed consequences of its operation have developed at the same time and in close connection with each other. Both have evolved out of an experimental method of procedure. At no time has he elaborated a theory for its own sake. This fact has sometimes been a disappointment to "intellectual" persons who have subconsciously got into the habit of depending on a certain paraphernalia of technical terminology. But the theory has never been carried beyond the needs of the procedure employed, nor beyond experimentally verified results. Employing a remarkably sensitive power of observation, he has noted the actual changes brought about in individuals in response to the means which he has employed. He has followed up these changes in their connections with the individual's habitual reflexes, noting the reactions due to the calling into play of established bad habits with even greater care than the more obvious beneficial consequences obtained. Every such undesirable response has been treated as setting a problem—namely, that of discovering some method of inhibiting these instinctive reactions and the feelings associated with them, and replacing them with acts which will give a basis for correct sensory appreciations. Every step in the process has been analyzed and formulated. Every changing condition and consequence, positive or negative, favorable or unfavorable, which is used as a means for developing the experimental procedure, has been still further developed. The use of this developed method has, of course, continuously afforded new material for observation and thorough analysis. To this process of simultaneous development of principles and consequences, used as means for testing each other, there is literally no end. As long as Alexander uses the method, it will be a process tending continually towards perfection. It will no more arrive at a stage of finished perfection than does any genuine experimental scientific procedure, with its theory and supporting facts. The most striking fact of Alexander's teaching is the sincerity and reserve with which he has never carried his formulation beyond the point of demonstrated facts.

It is obvious, accordingly, that the results obtained by Alexander's teaching stand on a totally different plane from those obtained under various systems which have great vogue until they are displaced by some other tide of fashion and publicity. Most of those who urge the claims of these systems point to "cures" and other specific phenomena as evidence that they are built upon correct principles. Even for patent medicines an abundance of testimonials can be adduced. But the theories and the concrete facts in these cases have no genuine connection with each other. Certain consequences, the "good" ones, are selected and held up for notice, whilst no attempt is made to find out what other consequences are taking place. The "good" ones are swallowed whole. There is no method by which it can be shown what consequences, if any, result from the principle invoked, or whether they are due to quite other causes.

But the essence of scientific method does not consist in taking consequences in gross; it consists precisely in the means by which consequences are followed up in detail. It consists in the processes by which the causes that are used to explain the consequences, or effects, can be concretely followed up to show that they actually produce these effects and no others. If, for instance, a chemist pointed, on the one hand, to a lot of concrete phenomena which had occurred after he had tried an experiment and, on the other hand, to a lot of general theories elaborately reasoned out, and then proceeded to assert that the two things were connected so that the theoretical principles accounted for the phenomena, he would meet only with ridicule. It would be clear that scientific method had not even been started; it would be clear that he was offering nothing but assertion.

Alexander has persistently discouraged the appeal to "cures" or any other form of remarkable phenomena. He has even discouraged keeping records of these cases. Yet, if he had not been so wholeheartedly devoted to working out a demonstration of a principle—a demonstration in the scientific sense of the word—he would readily have had his day of vogue as one of the miracle-mongers. He has also persistently held aloof from building up an imposing show of technical scientific terminology of physiology, anatomy, and psychology. Yet that course also would have been easy in itself, and a sure method of attracting a following. As a consequence of this sincerity and thoroughness—maintained in spite of great odds, without diversion to side-issues of fame and external success—Alexander has demonstrated a new scientific principle with respect to the control of human behavior, as important as any principle which has ever been discovered in the domain of external nature. Not only this, but his discovery is necessary to complete the discoveries made about non-human nature, if these discoveries and inventions are not to end by making us their servants and helpless tools.

A scientific person is quite aware that no matter how extensive and thorough is one's theoretical reasoning, and how definitely it points to a particular conclusion of fact, one is not entitled to assert the conclusion as a fact until one has actually observed the fact, until one's senses have been brought into play. With respect to distinctively human conduct, no one, before Alexander, has even considered just what kind of sensory observation is needed in order to test and work out theoretical principles. Much less have thinkers in this field ever evolved a technique for bringing the requisite sensory material under definite and usable control. Appeal to suggestion, to the unconscious and the subconscious, is in its very description an avoidance of this scientific task; the systems of purely physical exercise have equally neglected any consideration of the methods by which their faults are to be observed and analyzed.

Whenever the need has been dimly felt for some concrete check and realization of the meaning of our thoughts and judgments about ourselves and our conduct, we have fallen back, as Alexander so clearly points out in his writings, on our pre-existing sense of what is "right." But this signifies in the concrete only what we feel to be "familiar." And in so far as we have bad habits needing re-education, that which is familiar in our sense of ourselves and of our acts can only be a reflection of the bad psycho-physical habits that are operating within us. This is precisely as if a scientific person, who, by a process of reasoning, had been led to a belief in what we call the Copernican theory, were then to try to test this reasoning by appealing to precisely those observations, without any addition or alteration, which had led men to the Ptolemaic theory. Scientific advance manifestly depends on the discovery of conditions for making new observations, and on the re-making of old observations under different conditions; in other words, on methods of discovering why, as in the case of the scientist, we have had and relied upon observations which have led into error.

After studying over a period of years Alexander's method in actual operation, I would stake myself upon the fact that he has applied, to our ideas about ourselves and about our acts, exactly the same method of experimentation and of production of new sensory observations, as tests and means of developing thought, that have been the source of all progress in the physical sciences;

and if, in any other plan, any such use has been made of the sensory appreciation of our attitudes and acts, if in it there has been developed a technique for creating new sensory observations of ourselves, and if complete reliance has been placed upon these findings, I have never heard of it. In some plans there has been a direct appeal to "consciousness" (which merely registers bad conditions); in some, this consciousness has been neglected entirely and dependence placed instead upon bodily exercises, rectifications of posture, etc. But Alexander has found a method for detecting precisely the correlations between these two members, physical-mental of the same whole, and for creating a new sensory consciousness of new attitudes and habits. It is a discovery which makes whole all scientific discoveries and renders them available, not for our undoing, but for human use in promoting our constructive growth and happiness.

No one would deny that we ourselves enter as an agency into whatever is attempted and done by us. That is a truism. But the hardest thing to attend to is that which is closest to ourselves, that which is most constant and familiar. And this closest "something" is, precisely, ourselves, our own habits and ways of doing things as agencies in conditioning what is tried or done by us. Through modern science we have mastered to a wonderful extent the use of tools for accomplishing results upon and through other things. The result is all but a universal state of confusion, discontent, and strife. The one factor which is the primary tool in the use of all other tools—namely ourselves, our own psycho-physical disposition as the basic condition of our use of all agencies and energies—has not even been studied as the central instrumentality. Is it not highly probable that this failure explains why it is that, in mastering physical forces, we have ourselves been so largely mastered by them, until we find ourselves incompetent to direct the history and destiny of humanity?

Never before, I think, has there been such an acute consciousness of the failure of all external remedies as exists today, of the failure of all remedies and forces external to the individual. It is, however, one thing to teach the need of a return to the individual person as the ultimate agency in whatever humankind and society can collectively accomplish, to point out the necessity of straightening out this ultimate condition of whatever humanity in mass can attain. It is another thing to discover the concrete procedure by which this greatest of all tasks can be executed. And this indispensable thing is what Alexander has accomplished. The discovery could not have been made and the method of procedure perfected except by dealing with adults who were uncoordinated. But the method is not one of remedy; it is one of constructive education. Its proper field of application is with the young, with the growing generation, in order that they may come to possess as early as possible in life a correct standard of sensory appreciation and self-judgment. When once a reasonably adequate part of a new generation has become properly co-ordinated, we shall have assurance for the first time that men and women in the future will be able to stand on their own feet, equipped with satisfactory psycho-physical equilibrium to meet with readiness, confidence, and happiness—instead of with fear, confusion, and discontent—the buffetings and contingencies of their surroundings.

JOHN DEWEY

PART 1

Sensory Appreciation in Its Relation to Human Evolutionary Development

Sensory Appreciation in Its Relation to Human Evolutionary Development

Inadequacy of Subconscious Guidance and Control to Meet the Rapid Changes in Civilized Life

In *Man's Supreme Inheritance,* I contended that human beings cannot progress satisfactorily in civilization while they remain dependent on subconscious guidance (instinct). Dependence on this subconscious guidance in a rapidly changing civilization has resulted in the gradual development of defects in the use of the human organism.

(Note: The word "instinct" is used in this work to indicate established habits, inherited or developed. As I wrote in chapter 6 of *Man's Supreme Inheritance,* "I define instinct as the result of the accumulated subconscious experiences of humanity at all stages of our development, which continue with us until, singly or collectively, we reach the stage of conscious control.")

The effect of developing from a situation of slow, gradual change, to rapid environmental change under subconscious guidance could only be harmful; this is because many of our instincts survived their usefulness, while many new instincts which were developed quickly to meet new demands of civilization, proved unreliable. This unreliability grew until an observant minority noticed a most serious deterioration. Unfortunately they saw it as a physical deterioration only, and at this "psychological moment" in human development attempted to set it right by the adoption of "physical exercises."

Humanity has been and still is unable to adapt itself quickly enough to rapidly changing civilization. Results of the attempts we have made to adapt ourselves in the general use of the organism have been unsatisfactory and disappointing. One need only note the records of crime, unbalanced human thought, "trial-and-error" methods by leaders in their attempts to reform social conditions, industry, religion, politics, and education to be convinced of the comparative failure of our plan of life.

In order to understand humanity's comparative failure to adapt, it is necessary then to examine the evolutionary processes which existed in the primitive state and those which prevail now.

(At this point I would like to make clear that the term *psycho-physical* is used throughout my works to show the impossibility of separating "mental" and "physical" operations in our conception of the working of the human organism. I use the term *psycho-physical activity* to indicate all human manifestations, and *psycho-physical mechanism* to indicate the instrument which makes these manifestations possible.

Psycho-physical activity, however, does not always involve equal action of both, because history shows that at some stages in development there is a preponderance on the "physical" and at other stages on the "mental."

I am forced to use the terms "mental" and "physical" because there are no other words at present which adequately express psycho-physical activity. They cannot be separated. I use the word "mental" to mean processes which are not wholly "physical" and vice versa.)

Comparison of Evolutionary Processes in the Primitive and Civilized Stages

Firstly, it is important to remember that during the primitive stages of evolution, processes of development were very slow.

(Note: The word "evolution" is used to indicate all processes involved in the quickening of the potentialities of the creature at different stages of development, necessary to the success of his or her attempts to satisfy the needs of an ever-changing environment, and to reach a plane of constructive conscious control.)

Experts say it took millions of years of evolution to produce the primitive. Each later stage of development was the result of the experiences undergone by the creature. Years of repetition were probably needed to establish them as what is understood as instinct, because in subconscious development, continuous repetition is essential to establishing instinctive accuracy.

The law of self-preservation forced primitive humanity to use the mechanism to obtain food and avoid death. This process ensured an adequate and correct use of the psycho-physical organism *as a whole,* as well as an adequate and correct use *of the parts* of the organism.

Therefore at the start of civilization the creature functioned subconsciously in accordance with the dictates of instinct. It could meet the demands made upon it because the environment very rarely changed and when it did, it changed slowly.

But civilization called for an ever-improving standard in the development of the creature's potentialities. The rapid changes in the environment brought about more and yet more new needs, and the response to the stimuli resulting from these new needs had to be much quicker.

Furthermore—and this is all important—the demands made on the mental processes, comparatively unused at this time, increased very rapidly, while the demands made on the highly developed physical processes were destined to decrease, and their spheres of activity to become more and more limited with the advance of time. This shows that *it was essential that humanity should acquire a new way of directing and controlling the psycho-physical mechanism as a whole,* which in the primitive state had been up to a high standard of co-ordination in meeting the great "physical" demands of this way of life. This indicates that at some period of evolution the human being must have reached a psychological moment to pass from the subconscious to the conscious plane of control.

This change would have involved a knowledge of the *means* by which humanity would be able to command a conscious, reasoning direction and control of its psycho-physical mechanisms in all activity. With this knowledge we would have some chance of meeting satisfactorily the increasing demands of our ever-changing environment, and of commanding a continuous growth and development of the organism.

Unfortunately, the human being's ability to reason out the "means" of gaining its "ends" could not have been adequately established as a habit at this psychological moment in our development. If it had been, we would have realized that demands made upon us in the civilized state would be different from those in the primitive state.

(Note: Many readers of *Man's Supreme Inheritance* have asked for clarification of what I have called the "end-gaining" principle and the "means" principle. "End-gaining" involves a direct procedure by a person trying to reach the desired "end"; it depends upon subconscious guidance and control, leading in cases where there is malcoordination to unsatisfactory use of the mechanism and an increase in the defects already present. The "means," on the other hand, involves a reasoned consideration of the causes of the conditions present and an indirect procedure in trying to gain an "end." It involves conscious guidance and control and satisfactory use of the mechanism, which establishes the conditions essential to increasing the development of potentialities. Defects are not likely to be present in the organism. *In this connection I wish it to be understood that throughout this book, I use the term "conscious guidance and control" to indicate, primarily, a plane to be reached rather than a method of reaching it.*)

Humanity had not reached that stage of evolution that would have allowed the change from the subconscious to the conscious plane of control. Whilst, with the advance of civilization, conditions have continually changed and become more and more complex, our fundamental psycho-physical method of adapting to these changes has remained the same.

Complexity and Complications of Civilized Life

People generally accept that a growing complexity accompanied by stress and strain is the natural result of civilized life. They do not, however, recognize that this condition is the result of their own or others' ill-considered, end-gaining attempts to surmount the difficulties met during the progress of civilization. Thus, the egotism of the average human being is developed out of all proportion to the degree of successful endeavor that he or she can legitimately claim, and we are unlikely to awaken to our own shortcomings, unlikely to realize that *the fault, dear Brutus, is not in our stars but in ourselves.*

These prevailing conditions of stress and strain are harmful to the organism. If they increase as rapidly as in the past, then our reserves will be undermined and the most serious forms of organic disorder and kinesthetic perversion may be predicted. Indeed, we might say that a dangerous stage of perversion and delusion has already been reached, when attempts to solve all problems of life seem to call for complexity rather than simplicity. The most simple "means" become the most difficult. A well-known scientist having lessons with me had great difficulty with a simple, practical problem of psycho-mechanics and during a lesson said, "I know what is the matter with us all. This work of yours is too simple for us!"

In fact, the complexity needlessly introduced into the act of living in general is equaled only by the complexity which each individual builds up in attempts at accomplishment in specific spheres like education and self-instruction. The standard of efficiency in these spheres depends upon the individual's satisfactory use of his or her psycho-physical self. The imperfectly co-ordinated child or adult will not be likely to reach the standard of effective functioning of the co-ordinated one.

(Note: The word *co-ordination* is generally used in as narrow a sense as the words "relaxation," "re-adjustment," "re-education," etc. I wish to give a more comprehensive meaning to it as it is used in this work. I use it to convey co-ordination *on a general and not a specific basis*. Specific co-ordination of any part of the organism, such as the muscles of the arm or leg, may be done by a direct process, which will create new defects in the use of the organism, while others already present will become more pronounced. These defects will not occur if specific co-ordination is brought about through an indirect process, involving primarily the general co-ordination of the whole organism, an integrated condition.

The distinction between specific and general applies also to relaxation, re-education, and re-adjustment as used in this book because, in general re-education, specific defects are eradicated in process.)

In the uncoordinated child or adult, there are serious complications in the person's psycho-mechanics and difficulties are inevitable. On the other hand, in a co-ordinated person, the mechanical working of the structures of the organism is not complicated but complex—in the sense that, although there exists a large number of factors or means related to one another, the act of using them is simple. (Consider the complexity of the mechanisms of a car, but the simplicity of driving it.) Mechanical working does not become complicated until the mechanisms get out of order.

Take writing for example. In the uncoordinated child the act becomes a complicated procedure. Despite expert guidance from the teacher, the pupil does not possess the psycho-physical equipment which would enable him or her to take advantage of the instructions given. Each request from the teacher to do something and not to do something else causes a build-up of a series of psycho-physical acts towards the "end," the act of writing. The "end" may be gained, but the result as a *whole* will not be as satisfactory as it might be, because nothing has been done to re-educate the child on a general basis. The standard of success in the correct use of the fingers, wrist, and arm depends on the co-ordinated use of the mechanisms *in general.*

If the teacher gives correct instructions in the act of writing to a co-ordinated child, their assimilation would enable that child to reason out the "means" to accomplish the desired "end," which would be gained in an easy manner.

Recognition and Satisfaction of Essential Needs in Relation to Human Progress

Consideration of the psycho-physical "means" of making progress—urgently needed in human beings—may be helpful at this point. Satisfactory evolutionary progress demands a primary desire or need, which is the stimulus to the development of those psycho-physical potentialities required to meet the demands of the processes essential to meet that need. *The adequate development of these potentialities connotes a satisfactory standard of the co-ordinated use of the organism.*

A person satisfied with his or her position in evolution, with his or her ideas and opinions, will not have the desire or need to change conditions. Advancement, however, depends on discovering ideas, principles, ways of living, etc., new to the individual. Anyone who refuses to seek consciously for new experiences cannot expect any real advancement on the evolutionary plane.

In such a case, there is, for example, a narrow outlook, rigidity, dread of psycho-physical changes, lack of reasoning in guidance and control, all of which tend to prevent the person from conceiving, seeing, or accepting anything outside their present experiences. These experiences are the sum total of what they have inherited (represented by their race instincts) plus their comparatively limited experience in everyday life.

The establishment of such psycho-physical conditions means that perversions have built up subconsciously in the human being's everyday use of him or herself and sooner or later the person becomes aware of some shortcoming. It is probable that only one in twenty of these shortcomings ever reaches the conscious level, so the person continues to exist in a danger zone of sub-conscious psycho-physical shortcomings which impede progress at every turn.

Mind Wandering Recognized as a Shortcoming— Its Relation to Self-Preservation

The shortcoming that interferes most in the individual's attempts to learn something is one's inability to "keep one's mind" on the particular task in hand, whether in the activity of reading or in any other activity. This is commonly known as "mind-wandering."

What is mind-wandering? To answer this, the psycho-physical processes concerned with self-preservation must be considered. In the beginning of things, all growth and development must surely have come from a form of consciousness of need.

(Note: Many readers may not agree with me on this point, but it will be seen that all that is necessary to my argument is a recognition of the place of need, the requirement of a new way of linking up with the environment, so that the rest of my argument is not affected by belief or disbelief on this point.)

For the growth and development of the creature are and always have been associated with new experiences which involve new activities. These activities—the response to some stimulus or stimuli—result from the consciousness of some need inside or outside the organism, the presence and recognition of need being essential to the evolutionary process.

Recognition of need denotes a state of consciousness of a need. The primary activity which is a response to this involves new experiences in direction and control. The process of evolution depends upon the continuous repetition of such primary experiences, resulting in the establishment of a *use* (habit or instinct) and in the satisfaction of the need.

At one point in evolution, for instance, the development of a pair of eyes became a need. After the consciousness of this need arose, the growth of these organs may have occupied a thousand years or more and again have needed a conscious effort to open the eyelids and also to close them. Repetition of this conscious effort, week by week, month by month, and year by year may have caused this function of eyelids to become habitual and subconscious, and to develop to the wonderful standard of use now enjoyed by the human being.

(Note: I am quite aware, of course, that sensitiveness to light, likewise the eyes, developed long before there were any eyelids.)

There can be little doubt that self-preservation (in its broadest sense) was the most fundamental of the creature's needs. It needed to secure its own protection and preservation first, during its attempts to satisfy its specific needs.

The need for self-preservation called for that satisfactory direction and control which we find in wild animals and primitive people due to their circumstances, which would, in turn, enable the creature to respond to any stimulus by using the most satisfactory "means" to securing the essential "end," self-preservation.

The civilized person does not manifest anything like the marvelous accuracy in the use of the organism when it comes to self-preservation as does the wild animal or primitive person. This lack of control and direction shows itself, for example, in the sphere of learning something and learning to do something as the shortcoming of "mind-wandering."

There is a close connection between "mind-wandering" and the seriously weakened response to a stimulus to an act of self-preservation. To make this connection, consider the psycho-physical processes involved in these two shortcomings and you will realize that both are the same; that is, a lack of adequate direction and control in the broad sphere of self-preservation and in the specific sphere of learning something or learning to do something.

Whether in the sphere of self-preservation or of learning, a satisfactory response to a stimulus resulting from a need or wish depends on a satisfactory direction and control of the mechanism. The manifestation in our everyday life of an unsatisfactory response to a stimulus resulting from a need or a wish is called "mind-wandering."

Success in learning or learning to do depends upon satisfactory use of the psycho-physical mechanisms, which means attention to the "means" of doing something to gain a desired "end." Where a person's conception of the means to the end is satisfactory, mind-wandering will not occur.

On the other hand, failure to learn or learn to do something means there are defects in one's conception of the "means" to the act. The person will not gain the desired "end" because of defects in his or her psycho-physical mechanism, due to the inability to "keep the mind on" the work in hand.

Actually, defective use of the mechanism cannot be adequately described as "mind-wandering" because it is not only a misdirection of "mind," *but of the whole psycho-physical mechanism.* It is associated with an unreliable sense of feeling (sensory appreciation) and unsatisfactory direction and control, which has gradually weakened the human's response to stimuli in the sphere of self-preservation.

It is important to remember that the primitive human depended mainly on the sense of feeling, which was then comparatively reliable so that the direction and control of activities would be associated with an *increasing* response to the stimulus for self-preservation. The civilized human also depends on feeling (sensory-appreciation) but this is now harmfully unreliable, with an associated *weakening* response to the stimulus for self-preservation. This weakening condition of human psycho-physical direction and control has been brought about through dependence on subconscious guidance in our attempts to meet the demands of civilized existence. It is also due to reliance on instincts which have survived their usefulness, and harmful guidance of defective sense registers.

(Note: The fact that an individual happens to exhibit satisfactory direction and control in some particular activity does not confute this statement; indeed, only serves to strengthen it, as I hope to show in this book.

Too often in my work I have seen people who think that a psycho-physical experience is satisfactory, when I as an expert know it is not. It can be a delusive, harmful experience of feeling and thinking one is right when one is actually wrong. Later, when the person becomes dissatisfied, he or she does not attribute this dissatisfaction to their own psycho-physical experiences, but to "other people," "surroundings," "something wrong somewhere" —always believing the cause to be outside but not inside the organism.)

Experience follows experience in a person's activities, some satisfactory, but the majority unsatisfactory. Although we can be satisfied for the moment with results of attempted accomplishment, we then become dissatisfied again with the inconsistency; and our psycho-physical experiences do not make for confidence in our future attempts to cope with civilization.

Such conditions mean failure is almost certain to result, although the amount of time is spent which is considered necessary to ensure success. Eventually the person will wonder why, and this is of specific interest, because it will lead him or her to conclude that their failure is due to "mind-wandering."

Let us consider this in detail. Someone sets out to learn something or learn to do something, and "gives his mind" to his work. He soon discovers his "mind" is not "on his work," and is engaged in some other train of thought. Therefore, he makes a "specific effort" to "keep his mind on" the original task.

He has probably never considered whether he has the "means" of making a special effort within his control, and so, due to lack of this control his mind-wandering persists; after several repetitions, he concludes that the cause of his failure is his *inability* to keep his mind on what he is doing.

A psycho-physical disaster is indicated here, because the creature has reached that dangerous stage in the use of the mechanisms when the response to a stimulus arising from a need is ineffective, erratic, and confused.

The recognition of this serious inability to "keep the mind on" what one is doing has led to the general adoption of "concentration" as the cure for mind-wandering. Unfortunately, this remedy, as I will show later, is itself a harmful, delusive psycho-physical manifestation, adopted without consideration of its effect on the organism in general or of the psycho-physical processes involved in "learning to concentrate."

(Note: The recognition of mind-wandering long antedated the conception of concentration as its remedy. Fuller discussion on this will come in a later chapter. For now, I wish to point out that I do not object to "concentration" which implies a number of things going on, moving at the same time and converging on a common consequence, which is what happens in the normal child at play or the competent artisan or artist engrossed in his work, *and which simply implies a condition of co-ordination.* On the other hand I object to "concentration" which fixates on one thing, "bringing the mind to bear" on one object. Similarly, I object to the essential aim of education being the securing of "ends" by specific methods ("end-gaining") instead of being the due consideration of the "means" to an "end.")

Consideration of the Mechanism of the Psycho-Physical Organism in Relation to Learning and Learning To Do

As already indicated, in learning and learning to do, as in all psycho-physical acts, there is an important problem to be solved if we are to cope with the ever-increasing demands of an advancing civilization. The standard of functioning in the performance of any act depends on the *conception* which influences the direction and control of the mechanism. This matter of conception is all important in the understanding of what we wish to learn or learn to do, and of the psycho-physical activity involved.

Consider "learning" something. First, for every form of psycho-physical activity, there must be a stimulus. In considering the response to the stimulus, please remember not to separate the "mental" and the "physical." We cannot prove that the response to any stimulus is wholly "physical" or wholly "mental."

On the one hand, in performing "physical" acts the standard of functioning depends:

> (1) *upon the degree of correctness of the conception of the act to be performed;*
>
> (2) *upon the degree of co-ordinated use of the guiding and controlling directions, and of the mechanisms involved in carrying out the activities essential to the correct means of performance.*

On the other hand, in "mental" activity, the standard of functioning depends:

> (1) *upon the degree of reliability of the sensory guidance and direction in the use of the mechanisms involved in conveying the stimuli primarily responsible for the psycho-physical processes concerned with conception;*
>
> (2) *upon the standard of co-ordination reached in the use of the whole organism.*

If the highest standard of so-called physical functioning is to be reached, there must be *co-ordinated use of the muscular system, through co-ordinated direction and control by so-called mental processes, involving action and reaction in psycho-physical unity* and an adequate standard at all times of the vital functioning of the organism. This process works in reverse with regard to reaching the highest standard of so-called mental functioning.

(Note: When considering the vital functioning of the organism, we are all aware, for instance, that a sluggish liver does not allow the best use of the "mental" powers. Some people who have already reached a stage of liver or kidney disorder find their reasoning processes have become seriously impaired and those of remembering practically ruined. If this vital functioning is inadequate, the organism becomes poisoned with resulting interference with the ability to remember.)

No human activity, therefore, can be wholly "physical" or wholly "mental." *The standard of individual functioning is determined*

*by the standard of co-ordinated use of the organism in general,
which is, in turn, determined by the standard of co-ordinated use
of the psycho-physical processes involved.*

Psycho-physical activity is simply the response to stimuli received through the senses of sight, hearing, touch, feeling, etc. The
nature of the resulting conception and response is determined by
the standard of psycho-physical functioning present.

It then follows that *the process of conception, like all the other
forms of psycho-physical activity, is determined by our psycho-
physical condition at the time when the particular stimulus is
received.* We all know that a person's conception of, say their
financial affairs, or whatever, is different when in a "happy frame of
mind," from that when they have a "grouch." Also the conception
as to the outcome of a disaster or piece of good fortune in life will
be quite different in a healthy person from an unhealthy one.

Influence of Sensory Appreciation upon Conception
in All Psycho-Physical Activity

This dependence of the process of conception on the general
psycho-physical condition is of paramount importance. If all
"mental" processes are mainly the result of sensory experience, it
will be obvious that in our conception of *how* to use the different
parts of the mechanism in everyday acts *we are influenced chiefly
by sensory processes* (feeling). Thus, we may receive a stimulus
through something we hear or touch, for example; in every case
the nature of our response, *whether it be an actual movement, an
emotion, or an opinion,* will depend on the associated activity,
(reaction and action) of the processes of conception and sensory
and other mechanisms responsible for the "feeling" which we
experience. This associated activity is referred to throughout
my work as *sensory appreciation.*

Sensory Appreciation

This sensory appreciation is the factor on which the baby, like the animal, depends for guidance in its first subconscious attempts to use its mechanism, the child's success depending on the degree of reliability of his or her sensory appreciation. I assert that any defects in children at a very early age, even in attempts at crawling, walking, etc., are present because the child's instinctive processes are unreliable. It is my purpose throughout this book to prove this. Also I wish to show that in cases where instinctive processes are unreliable we must restore the sensory appreciation to an adequate level.

A comprehensive understanding of sensory appreciation, of its enormous influence for good or bad in human development and its future bearing on the progress of humankind, is, therefore, of the greatest importance to all, but especially to those interested in education, both in our schools and in the broadest sense of the word.

Sensory appreciation has much wider significance than is generally attributed to it. It includes, at the very least, experiences conveyed through sight, hearing, touch, feeling, equilibrium, movement, etc., which are responsible for psycho-physical action and reaction.

In moving a limb or any other movement, we are guided mainly by sensory appreciation, our sense of feeling. This applies to testing the texture of a piece of cloth with the fingers or to the gauging of size, weight, or distance, etc.—in fact to the use of the "physical" mechanisms in any activity of life.

The Human and the Inanimate Machine Compared and Contrasted

The function of sensory appreciation will be clear if we consider the human organism as an animate machine, compared to an inanimate machine.

In the inanimate machine, the controlling mechanism is limited by the fixed nature of its own make-up and by its fixed conditions in other mechanisms, without which it could not operate.

In the human organism, the controlling mechanism is a wonderful psycho-physical process (the all-important difference) by which an almost unlimited use of the different parts may be brought about, so that at one moment a correct use and at another moment an incorrect use may be commanded. This psycho-physical process is that essential factor in satisfactory human development which we call sensory appreciation. Our ability to reach our maximum potential depends on the standard of its reliability.

Unreliable Sensory Appreciation a Universal Defect

The sensory appreciation of the people of our time is unreliable and in the great majority, positively delusive. Readers of *Man's Supreme Inheritance* will probably be convinced of this.

Example: Take a man who persistently puts his head back whenever he attempts to move his shoulders back. Ask him to put his head forward and keep his shoulders still; he will move his shoulders also. Ask him then to put his head forward while the teacher holds his shoulders still; he will, in practically every instance, put his head back.

Example: Ask a pupil to turn his toes out and, in my experience, instead of taking his body weight on his heels, he takes it on the balls of his feet and still tries to move the front parts outwards, or he moves the heels towards one another, instead of turning out the toes. Point this out to the pupil and he, as if aware of the sensory delusion, at once looks down at his feet to *see* how to move them correctly.

Example: Few people can open the mouth without putting the head back, as though lifting the upper jaw away from the lower. They do not realize that subconscious processes operate continuously to keep the mouth closed. Consequently the first thing to do is stop these processes and allow the jaw to drop.

When I ask a pupil to allow me to move her jaw she usually increases instinctively the tension that keeps the lower jaw in place. An enormous amount of energy is wasted in these constant, irrational tensions.

Many who are shown that the sensory appreciation of most modern people is more or less unreliable, become unusually disturbed, especially when they realize that this fundamental factor in human activity has been practically ignored by our experts and leaders in educational and other spheres in their efforts to effect reforms in the civilizing plan. This is indeed a fearful fact to ask the ordinary human being to face. When I have been forced to impress it on my pupils, I have read in their faces the different ideas, opinions, and feelings evoked by my statement. Very often they have looked upon me almost as an enemy.

For example, I was discussing this with a friend who at once denied that our sensory appreciation was unreliable and asked, "Why should Nature *permit* us to go wrong in such an essential?" I agreed to answer if he could tell me why Nature *should* prevent us from going wrong, seeing that in the process of our development in civilization even the simplest fundamentals of Nature have been ignored. My original statement had caused an emotional reaction to a shock in my friend and not a reasoning one. He admitted later that until I brought the matter up he had never considered this question of unreliable sensory appreciation, and yet had disagreed with someone who had studied it for thirty years and taught it for twenty-five. The truth is, we have not given sufficient consideration to this essential matter and we presume, in the usual subconscious way, that as a matter of course, our sensory appreciation must be reliable.

Consideration of Three Stages of Human Development in Relation to Deterioration of Sensory Appreciation

I will now attempt to give certain facts regarding stages in the evolution of the human being, when psycho-physical conditions became present which made for the gradual deterioration of sensory appreciation, indicating possible causes of such deterioration. I will confine this consideration to three stages:

(1) the stage when we were guided mainly by sensory appreciation;

(2) the stage when we were developing the ability to inhibit in

specific spheres and were still "physically fit";

(3) the stage when we had still further developed the ability to inhibit in specific spheres, but had recognized a lower standard of "physical" fitness which needed a remedy.

STAGE 1: UNCIVILIZED STAGE
Standard of Sensory Appreciation Reliable and Satisfactory Conditions Maintained

We are all aware of the higher standard of sensory appreciation in the uncivilized as compared with the civilized state. In this first stage, the satisfactory condition in the primitive person was maintained by the constant use of the mechanisms in the limited spheres of activity concerned with obtaining food, drink, and shelter, and with preserving life from human and other enemies. Subconscious guidance satisfactorily met his or her needs. These people were unaware, that is, of the *means* by which they controlled their mechanisms in their everyday activities, and this unawareness did not matter at this stage.

The reason for this is that the standard of co-ordination and sensory appreciation was very high and uncivilized existence did not call for continual adaptation to rapid changes. In fact this "physical" condition of the primitive at that period had reached an excellent state. For if we are justified in believing that the two-footed upright creature inherited from its four-footed predecessor a well-developed, healthy organism, we may assume that it reached the human stage in a relatively high state of health.

(Note: This does not exclude the possibility of the creature's experiencing occasional aches and pains or even suffering specific diseases; but excluding this, the usual level was a normal one. It is significant that primitive humans always think of disease after the analogy of wounds from arrows, stone bruises, etc.—that is, as coming specifically from out-side—and the technique of the medicine man is to drive out the foreign substances that have come in; if he sweats the patient, for instance, it is to expel some foreign substance.)

During slow growth over thousands of years, the human being built up a use and development on the so-called physical side in an environment which rarely changed—and if it did, then only gradually—so that his or her activities involved the daily repetition of the same acts, whose standard of difficulty remained about the same.

But on the so-called mental side his use and development had been comparatively limited in the daily tasks of hunting for food—using instinct which was as sure a guide as that of the prey.

With this relatively high "physical" standard and the associated development of the organism in general, the experience of ill-health must have been small. If someone did get ill, there can be little doubt that they would use some root or herb which they knew would cure them.

(Note: Thus we see that the habit of "taking something" for an ill had a very early origin. This habit led to the coming of the medicine man. For one of the first channels we humans would direct our developing intelligence into would be the discovery of the means of remedying our physical ill. This was bound to produce men and women who would devote themselves exclusively to the study of such ills and their remedies.)

This would be a subconscious reaction to the stimulus of the sense of ill-being, just as we had a reaction to the stimulus of hunger, that is, to hunt for food. *As long as we possessed a mechanical organism which worked accurately, instinctive procedure served our purpose.*

The "specific" cure was in keeping with natural requirements. Just as instinct guided us in daily life when we were well, it would guide us when we were ill to the necessary specific remedy, through the only part of our organism which was as yet highly developed, namely, sensory appreciation. This means that our sense of taste and smell would be working in co-ordination with our stomach and digestive processes.

So, whether well or ill, our instinct was reliable in the slowly

changing routine of daily life, so that, because of instinct's association with reliable sensory appreciation, we would have no need of
recourse to the higher directive processes.

STAGE 2: EARLY CIVILIZING STAGE
*Development of Reasoning Inhibition and the
Beginning of the End of the Dominance of Instinct
as a Controlling Factor*

As time went on, reasoning came more and more to illumine the
creature's dull and limited existence, shown by the fact that it
began to construct crude weapons and shelters. These reasoning
processes were destined to grow and develop through the myriad
operations of evolutionary building involved in the new and
diverse experiences concerned with our progress towards a higher
plane. Gradually, through reasoning inhibition, we were able,
within certain well-defined limits, to master or modify the desires
and tendencies of that sensory mechanism on which up to then
we had depended entirely for judgment and direction.

The development of these reasoning processes distinguished
primitive humanity from the lower animals, but more importantly,
it marked the "beginning of the end" of the dominance of instinct
as a controlling factor in human activity: from this period onwards,
humans could no longer live and move satisfactorily by subconscious guidance alone.

How did these reasoning processes work in this new situation?
In emerging from the primitive state, environmental changes
were at first slow and gradual, and the consequent demands on our
newly developing reasoning would have been correspondingly
light. Then, as civilization advanced with increasing rapidity,
humans must have been placed more and more in new and untried
situations, which would demand an increasing use of our reasoning powers. This was exactly the opposite of the earlier primitive
situation where conditions called for a relatively higher development on the "physical" than on the "mental" side. It is conceivable,
therefore, that the new civilized conditions called for a rapid

increase in our "mental" powers. There is little doubt that at this stage we had not become dissatisfied with the results of this changing process, and we continued to receive from inside and outside more stimuli to "mental" than to "physical" activities. "Mental" stimuli became more frequent and new situations made more demands on us to deal with them, thus further developing our reasoning processes in the constant inhibition of our natural desires, so as to enable us to meet the demands of a young and developing society.

Humanity had left its familiar environment behind. As the path of our new experiences opened out, we were confronted with one of the greatest difficulties yet encountered in our evolutionary progress, namely, that of adapting quickly to an ever more rapidly changing environment which entailed new psycho-physical experiences.

And we did adapt to these new conditions while our sensory appreciation was still more or less reliable, else we could not have survived; but it was only in the same way that we had always survived, that is, by trusting blindly to subconscious instinct. Thus, it seems that early in our civilized career, we presumed subconsciously that we were equipped in every way for any new procedure in life, such as sawing, plowing, chopping, etc., and even, in time, for occupations which entailed working in cramped and difficult conditions.

At this early stage we were justified in believing that, faced with any new task, we could probably carry it out with impunity. Nothing had so far occurred to make us suspect that our sensory appreciation was not reliable, or our co-ordination unsatisfactory, or that in adapting our mechanism to new activities in a *specific way* we might be injuring them in a *general way,* which would gradually lead to a general deterioration. The same subconscious guidance through our sensory appreciation which we had relied on in the past, was relied on for all the new and varied occupations of civilization.

This shows that although we had developed our reasoning

processes to some extent in, for example, the invention of crude implements, we did not go on to apply them to the directing of our psycho-physical mechanisms in the use of ourself in everyday activities. With our reasoning processes thus limited in their use, and no awareness, as yet, of any sense of physical shortcoming, it is most unlikely that we could have received even a slight subconscious hint that our instinct would be affected in the new surroundings and experiences of civilization. Neither did we suspect that we could ever lose a fraction of the satisfactory "physical" use which the race had enjoyed for countless ages, which was then our inheritance, and which we never doubted we would hand down to our successors for all time.

Had we reasoned the matter out, we would have realized that many of our instincts were being used less and less in the old ways and consequently were becoming less reliable. *It would then have been obvious that in order to meet satisfactorily the requirements of our new and changing environment, we must employ new guidance and direction, and that, in order to build up this new guidance with the rapidity that our necessities demanded, we must call on reasoning to supersede instinct (the co-worker of slow development) in the use of our psycho-physical mechanisms. In other words, we would have realized that our primitive psycho-physical equipment must pass from the subconscious to the conscious plane of guidance and direction.*

Centuries passed, bringing an increasing scope for the use of humanity's reasoning processes. Unfortunately, we confined this to the consideration of the relation of "cause and effect," "means and ends," in connection with our activities in the outside world, both social and physical. We failed to apply the same consideration to our use of the psycho-physical organism, which was being gradually interfered with.

The results of the failure of humanity's instincts to meet the new demands of civilization would not show themselves all at once. It is reasonable to suppose that, as humans emerged from the primitive state, their instinct was still working satisfactorily

and that there was little need for "cures" because of their comparatively high standard of health. Up to then the so-called physical self
was more highly developed and had been the controlling factor in
their activities. It is almost beyond human power today to realize
that the experiences of millions of years had gone into the building-up of this so-called physical development. The experiences
humanity had gained on the so-called mental side were infinitesimal in comparison.

From now on, this restless, inquisitive creature possessing
wonderful potentialities and developing much faster on the
"mental" than the "physical" side, continued to progress in civilization, with ever-increasing speed. But its race instincts had
not equipped it for such a sudden psycho-physical rush, such a
tremendous overbalancing on the "mental" side; so that we arrived
at the new stage breathless, dazed, at a loss, as it were, from the
lack of the graduated psycho-physical experiences which had been
part and parcel of our earlier growth.

(Note: This indicates (1) that conscious reasoned psycho-
physical activity must replace subconscious guidance in cop-
ing with civilization; (2) that these changes must be made
more quickly than before to meet this demand satisfactorily;
and (3) that, with the passing of time, there will be a corresponding need for improvement in the sphere of psycho-
physical activity.

In short, the fundamental difficulty arises from the
following facts. Uncivilized humanity relied on subconscious
control, and probably hundreds of years were spent making
simple changes, because subconscious activity is very slow
to respond to the need for change. Civilized humanity still
relies on subconscious guidance just as it did when uncivilized—the tragedy of civilization. Although we have remained satisfied with the form of direction and control used
to bring about change, we have become dissatisfied with the
time taken to make the changes. It is humanity's supreme
civilizing blunder that we have failed to realize in practice

that rapid changes in civilization call for a corresponding quickening in our use of the psycho-physical mechanisms, possible only on a plane of constructive conscious control.)

STAGE 3: LATER CIVILIZING STAGE
Recognition of a Serious Shortcoming Which Was Called Physical Deterioration

There came, at last, a time in the history of humanity when a number of people became aware of a certain serious shortcoming. The adoption of "physical exercises" as a remedy is proof that they recognized this shortcoming as a "physical" deterioration. This shortcoming and general undermining of well-being was to accompany us from then onwards to the present time.

Our error was that we did not recognize that this was not a "physical" shortcoming only, but that we had reached a psychological moment in our development: the time had come for us to come into our great inheritance, that is, to pass from the subconscious to the conscious use of our psycho-physical mechanisms.

There certainly was a recognition of so-called physical deterioration unlike any previously recognized experience of humankind. There may even have also been a sense of gain through the increased use and development of the so-called mental processes. But the point I wish to make clear is that, with this unequal development, there had been an inadequate co-ordinating process at work that has continued, with but few exceptions, in human beings to the present day. The process of civilization tended to widen the scope for "mental" development and to narrow it for "physical" activities, and this gradual deterioration on the "physical" side caused an accompanying deterioration in our sensory appreciation. We must remember in relation to this, that, because of the interrelation and interdependence of the mechanisms and potentialities of the organism in life, any deterioration on the "physical" side must eventually seriously affect the "mental" side. Enlargement of the spheres of so-called mental activity does not necessarily denote a growth of healthy "mental" activity.

(Note: "Mental" growth continued even after "physical" deterioration had been recognized. One might say that one limb (mental) of the tree grew at such a terrific pace that the tree overbalanced, seriously disturbing the roots responsible for its equilibrium.)

This has been proved, for instance, by the events of 1914–1918. In fact, the process of civilization has gone hand in hand with harmful interference of those co-ordinating processes on which humanity's satisfactory psycho-physical growth depends.

From the start of civilization, then, human growth on this subconscious basis was bound to be uneven and unbalanced. This unbalanced development marked the beginning of the interference with our co-ordinated use of the mechanism as a whole, and particularly with those muscular co-ordinations so essential to "physical" well-being.

Interference with the Co-ordinated Use of the Psycho-Physical Mechanism and an Associated Lowering of the Standard of Sensory Appreciation

In the primitive state, instinctive guidance was associated with co-ordinated use of the human mechanism and reliable sensory appreciation. This old instinctive guidance gradually lost its usefulness under the new conditions and became more or less impaired, but the same implicit reliance was placed on it as in our uncivilized days. The inevitable result was an interference in co-ordination and a lowering of the standard of sensory appreciation. The harm was intensified because we continued to depend on our ever deteriorating sense of feeling, so that we have come to represent perhaps the most imperfectly co-ordinated type of human ever known.

It is, therefore, easy to understand how this gradual interference and deterioration at last reached a point where the need for a remedy became very urgent and where humanity had to face a situation that now demanded a *quick* response. The problem was further complicated by the fact that we were badly co-ordinated, and had acquired, by reason of the speed with which our experiences had been gained, the habit of acting in a certain confident, almost reckless, way to stimuli.

Thus, when the urgent call for a remedy arose, it caused great confusion accompanied by hasty decision-taking because humanity had already reached such an advanced stage of psycho-physical malcoordination. These experiences repeated indefinitely: (1) the increasing sense of shortcoming, (2) the urgent S.O.S. call for a remedy, and (3) the hurried haphazard response, showing that the disturbed condition involved is not conducive to the employment of the reasoning processes.

(Note: Under these conditions unreliable lines of communication can become established, with the associated unsatisfactory psycho-physical actions and reactions. These will have that general effect on the kinesthesia which leads in time to the fixed habit or phobia so common today and so wrongly called nerves [anxiety or stress—ed.] or neurasthenia.)

We remember Carlyle's reaction, who, on hearing of his friend's illness, rushed off with a bottle of medicine, without even knowing what was ailing him. If a man of such attainments, living in a so-called advanced civilization, acted at a psychological moment in such an unreasoning way, it is not surprising that the subconsciously-guided human of an earlier period rushed to find a "cure" for his deterioration in the same unreasoning way. As far as we can judge, he subconsciously adopted the form of "cure" to which instinct had prompted his ancestors in the past. But this form of "cure" was no longer suited to his life circumstances, because of the ever-changing demands of civilization.

Because primitive humanity, then, had always sought a *specific* "cure," instinctively choosing a particular root or berry to heal some specific pain or hurt, we now followed the same instinct to deal with our problems *specifically*. Recognizing that our muscular development was deteriorating, we decided that our loss of health was *due* to this deterioration alone—and not to a deterioration of the general psycho-physical adjustment of our organism with a misplacement of vital organs and viscera, causing serious pressure and irritation, and causing the disagreeable and alarming symptoms.

(Note: Unfortunately, this narrow view is still held by most physiologists and anatomists. One need only watch the movements of many who are experts in these subjects to realize the futility of their knowledge from a practical point of view. For the knowledge of the ordinary anatomical and physiological workings of specific muscles does not enable any person to re-educate or co-ordinate them on a general basis in the acts of everyday life, *and it is on this basis of common sense and practice that the value of any knowledge or principle must be judged.*)

Specific Remedy Chosen to Counteract a General Malcondition

Humanity concluded that its general shortcomings were due to specific muscular shortcomings. This narrow, erroneous conception led directly to the idea of muscle development by means of *specific* exercises, to be performed at *specific* times, to develop *specific* muscles. Evidently, this process could not satisfactorily stop our *general* deterioration.

Let us consider, for example, the "weight-lifting-conception," a crude remedy indeed, well in keeping with the stage of evolution in which instinct had become impaired and the reasoning processes were, as yet, employed only in limited spheres. (In *Man's Supreme Inheritance*, I have pointed out that these muscle-building exercises are still being gradually modified.) Weight-lifting was superseded by a crude form of gymnasium where strenuous exercise was performed. These primitive mechanical exercises were, in turn, succeeded by less strenuous ones, and then again by an increasing number of muscle-building machines which became the vogue. It was evident that the results were unsatisfactory, and that psycho-physical deterioration was still continuing. Changes were made. Swedish drill became the fashion, exercisers and dumbbells were used in muscle-tensing movements of all kinds. Experiences concerned with posture, calisthenics, plastic dancing, deep breathing, "Daily Dozens," and other specific methods were also used but found unsatisfactory. The search for the "great unknown or unrecognized" still continues.

Another set of people came to think that civilization was never meant as a way of life, and feel that a "return to Nature" or "the simple life" is the remedy. But the idea of a civilized person trying to return to the environment of our prehistoric ancestors would make one laugh, were it not for the tragedy involved in a conception which is so uncomplimentary to our intellectual pride.

Certain Errors of Judgment in the Choice of "Physical Exercises" as a Remedy for a Fundamental Shortcoming

I wish to emphasize that, throughout our long search for the remedy for our deterioration, we overlooked, and still do today, certain most important factors. Firstly, we overlooked the fact that our sensory mechanism was no longer registering accurately and that we could not, therefore, continue to rely entirely on feeling to guide us. It is clearly unreasonable to expect "physical exercises," of whatever kind, to bring about any lasting, fundamental improvement, when in performing them, the person has to *depend on the guidance of the very thing which has led to the condition we wish to remedy—our delusive sensory appreciation.* Furthermore, performing "physical exercises" would lead to the actual development of one's original malcoordinated condition, and to some new and very baffling psycho-physical problems in oneself.

(Note: In the second part of this book, I will deal with some of these problems as they occur in education and in other areas of life.)

These problems arose and have since then become increasingly complicated. Although they are not entirely overlooked today, their real significance is still almost entirely misunderstood. Most people do not realize that humans are propelling an already maladjusted and damaged mechanism along the difficult road of modern life, and, in doing so, still relying on imperfect and some-times delusive sensory appreciation for guidance.

Secondly, in adopting "physical exercises" as a remedy, we did not consider that our body is a very delicate and highly co-ordinated piece of machinery, so that many more causes other than muscular weakness may have contributed to our deteriora-tion. Further, that the exercises were not correlated in any way to the needs of our organism, either in the practical activities of life or during rest periods, which are such an important part of the daily round (a point constantly overlooked by "physical culture" enthusiasts).

If we ask ourselves why earlier people overlooked these im-portant points, the answer may throw light on many of our own problems at the present time. It was undoubtedly because they were seeking a method of "cure," and not prevention. In the terms of my thesis, their attention was fixed on the "end" they were seeking ("physical" amelioration), not on the reasonable *means* of securing that "end."

They did not see that their deterioration was accompanied by an interference with the general adjustment of the organism and was merely the symptom of some failure in the working of his machin-ery, *and that the whole machine would need to be re-adjusted before it could work co-ordinatedly once more.*

If they had seen this, they would have dealt with it like any other machine—their watch, for instance—if it was not working. For, of course, if a watch were out of order, they would not trust its accuracy if they wanted to catch a train. And if they did not know how to fix it, they would not start to repair it at random, but rather send it to an expert who did know. Part of the watchmaker's advice would probably be a periodic overhaul, for example, *as a preventive measure.* By this means a reasonable effort would be made to *prevent* the watch from going wrong again.

(Note: We must again note the difference between human and inanimate machinery. The human machine, when in a state of co-ordinated and adequate use, commands in itself the power of growth and development in each part of the muscular mechanism. The condition equivalent to "wear" in inanimate machinery may be prevented from becoming present in the human being by Nature's method of supply and repair under right conditions in the matter of used and wasted tissue.)

It is no surprise, however, that humanity did not reason in the same way about its own mechanism. Our reasoning processes had not been employed to anywhere near the same degree with regard to our own mechanism, as they had been with the mechanisms of external nature. We thought we had discovered a "physical" defect for which we must find a remedy: any other possible consideration was shut off, whether of the causes of the "physical" deterioration, or of the psycho-physical principles involved, or of the *"means"* of securing the desired "end" (remedy). The decision was, therefore, a subconscious, not a conscious, reasoning one. A different result could hardly be expected at this early stage of human development, seeing that even today, in the twentieth century, the problem of psycho-physical unfitness is met with the same primeval "remedy" outlook, both in theory and practice.

Conscious Reasoning Processes Applied in Connection with Outside Activities But Not in Connection with the Psycho-Physical Organism

The stubborn but unpleasant fact must be faced: Although we have reasoned out the "means" of controlling the different forces we have discovered in the outside world, we have not applied this reasoning principle where our own organism is concerned. We have left this masterpiece of psycho-physical machinery, more subtle, more delicate in its workings than the most intricate man-made machine, to the subconscious guidance of our sensory appreciation, unaware that this sensory appreciation is becoming more and more unreliable with the boasted advance of civilization.

(Note: It is well known that a passion for mechanics exists among boys of our time. How very easy it would be to turn this desire towards an understanding of their own mechanisms!)

Is it not a sacrilege that during the past two thousand years of civilization the human organism has been used on a subconscious and unreasoned plan, so that defects and distortions have become established? This wonderful machinery has been harmfully interfered with, resulting in a lowered standard of general functioning.

There was a time when the body and limbs of the human being were an inspiration to sculptor and painter, a joy to look on as a thing of beauty and symmetry. In our time, however, the organisms of the vast majority of people are more or less maladjusted and unsymmetrical. Awkwardness and ungainliness have superseded grace and poetry of motion, shapely limbs have become misshapen, and the psycho-physical mechanisms are employed not to advantage but to disadvantage.

To sum up, we have seen how, in choosing "physical exercises" as a remedy for physical deterioration, people overlooked certain important facts. Firstly, they failed to recognize that sensory appreciation was no longer a reliable guide. Secondly, they did not think of the body as a co-ordinated whole, and were therefore misled into choosing a specific remedy instead of using *preventive principles*. Above all, they did not apply the one great principle on which I claim satisfactory progress in civilization depends— the principle of *thinking out the reasonable means of achieving a certain end*, instead of the old subconscious way of working blindly for an immediate "end."

We can now understand that a fundamental process has been, and continues to be established today, in the great majority of people who, at certain psychological moments, still act in the same way as their forbears of the Dark Ages. When faced with problems, they still work subconsciously for their immediate "ends" ("cure" idea), instead of first thinking out the reasonable *means* of achieving their "ends" (prevention idea).

It is true that some modification is going on here and there. A small minority of people are actually attempting to analyze their own and others' cases, where illness and imperfections are concerned. But, as I will show later, they are all attempting to make "cures" by means of *specific* remedy, instead of dealing with each problem on a *general* basis.

This applies equally to the various forms of so-called mental healing, including Christian Science, Auto-suggestion, New Thought, etc. These are simply reactions from the earlier idea of "physical culture," reactions from one extreme to another. Indeed, in most of our attempts at progress on a subconscious plane, we tend to move from one extreme to the other, until Nature does something to make us pause. We then, perhaps, retrace our steps, only to start off just as blindly in another direction until we reach another extreme (a process which amounts to over-compensation). Nature then forces us once more to halt. This is like a man lost in the wild, who wanders in a circle, failing to observe the signs, and finds himself back where he started. It is this habit of rushing from one extreme to the other, this tendency to take the narrow and treacherous sidetracks instead of the great, broad, midway path, that has caused our plan of civilization to be a comparative failure.

Harmful Concepts of Division of the Psycho-Physical Organism

There is one more aspect of my case which epitomizes all the errors which we humans have made in our efforts to cope with the problems of civilization while relying on subconscious guidance. In the adoption of "physical exercises" and of various methods of "mental healing," we have made an arbitrary attempt to separate the psycho-physical organism into body, mind and soul.

(Note: The unity of human potentialities on which I base my philosophy and practice, has, up till now, been represented as "body," "body and mind," or "body, mind, and soul." These words are in common use. Now we do know something tangible about the body, but what do we really know about "soul" or "mind"? Yet phrases such as to "hold in mind," to "keep the mind on," "improving the mind," "developing the mind," etc., are in continual use. We also talk of "mental" attitude, "mental" habits, "mental" control, etc.

I have argued in *Man's Supreme Inheritance* and in this book, that harmful results will follow the efforts of people beset with unreliable sensory appreciation, when they try to follow out written or spoken instructions, with the aim of eradicating defects in the use of their psycho-physical mechanisms. It is possible to acquire some knowledge of the working of these mechanisms; if, then, harmful results can follow attempts at improvement in this area where tangible knowledge can be acquired, how much more harm can be done in attempting to follow out such specific instructions as to "hold something in mind" or "keep the mind" on something, when we have no tangible knowledge of the working of what we call "mind." Then, when we reach the point where we can suggest the possibility of "developing" or "making" a "mind," we are so far removed from concrete realization of facts as to have reached the borderland of mysticism. Humanity's efforts during its development give proof of the harm done whenever we attempt to respond to a stimulus arising from our conception of a phrase which represents intangible phenomena. How can this be otherwise? How can we come to possess any tangible "means" by which we can gain an intangible "end"? This is why I give so many concrete illustrations in my books. Here we have something demonstrable in simple, practical procedures, and free from those intangible phenomena which are too often inseparable from what is known as "mental" or "spiritual" discussion.

If it were not for the worldwide tragedy of it all, one could be almost amused at those who attempt to pierce the veil of the "beyond" while they are still ignorant of discoverable potentialities within their grasp. Is it not reasonable to assume that knowledge of the "means" of continuously developing these potentialities should be the stepping stone to satisfactory activities on other planes of life? Surely humankind should at least come into the great earthly inheritance—the conscious plane of evolution—before time and energy are devoted to those fields of speculation and doubt in connection with the "undiscover'd country from whose bourn no traveller returns.")

To separate any organism into parts and then expect it to function satisfactorily is an unreasoned proposition, as unreasoned as it would be to expect the best results from any other machine by separating the gear mechanism, for instance, from the explosive and steering mechanism. It is probable that this unreasoned conception had its origin in that confused condition generally associated with fear, in some form or other. The confused state into which humanity was thrown in its first attempts to find a "cure" for its deterioration was naturally linked up to its original fears. For fear has been humanity's constant companion from the earliest times, and whether a healthy or an unhealthy fear, it was a form of illness for which the lowly developed creature could not find a "cure." The primary law that one creature should feed on another, the shock of new experiences, and the ignorance of the simple laws of Nature were responsible for this. There was no escape. Every creature lived in constant expectation of an attack by an enemy. The canary whose great, great, great, grandparents were caged birds, still looks from side to side with anxious rapidity after picking up each seed, just like the earliest of its kind.

Imagine a primitive man's first reaction to thunder and lightning, when his very existence depended on *a proper response to the stimulus of fear.* His reaction to such fears was to seek refuge in the supernatural. Indeed, civilized men who ridicule the practice of prayer, have been known to kneel and pray instinctively in circumstances such as a shipwreck. In these cases, fear overrules their convictions, primitive subconsciousness holds sway, and they probably fall to their knees without knowing it.

So it would be with a primitive man. Terrified by the thunder and lightning, he would drop down, hide his face in his hands, mumbling, incoherently perhaps, to "something." After the storm when his fear subsided, it is conceivable that he would think that the first object, tree or stone, to meet his terrified gaze was the power which saved him from an awful fate. Worship of wooden and stone images probably developed from these experiences.

Let us pass over the intervening stages and go on to consider how this fear manifests itself in the modern Christian era. Here we find that humanity's fears lessened in the case of thunder and lightning and of other terrors with which we had now become familiar, but are no less acute in new and unfamiliar spheres. And beyond this original fear of the unknown, a new form of fear had come upon us, through the one-sided development of our organism. For unbalanced psycho-physical development connotes unsatisfactory equilibrium in all spheres, and unsatisfactory equilibrium is always associated with fear. Since entering into the civilized state, humanity had been developing more rapidly on the "mental" side while deteriorating on the "physical." We had, therefore, been building up two forces within us—two separate entities almost—the one working against the other. The conflicting demands of these two "separate entities" has interfered with our equilibrium and produced in us the condition of inward fear, a condition which today is too often called "nerves" ["anxiety," "stress" —ed.].

(Note: The presence of fear always means a condition of conflict. The person who is inwardly afraid puts on an outward show of bravery by an assumed manner. Similarly, it is doubtless this inward fear which causes in nations a mania for carrying arms and for the massed attack in accordance with their horde instinct.)

This new fear—*actually a fear of himself*—gradually developed until it was recognized as an urgent problem. In our solution of this problem, we are faced with a most harmful conception when considered in relation to our evolutionary progress: this conception being the separation of the organism into soul, mind, and body. We attempted to develop each of these three "parts" specifically, and even made a "class-distinction," as it were, between them—a procedure which was a reversion to "habit of thought" associated with other spheres. Surely, even believing in this separation, our knowledge of the process of Nature indicates the place which the body should hold in order of importance.

The argument so far is, that:

(1) Rules of moral, social, and other conduct already established at the period designated the Christian era were the result of human conceptions.

(2) The human beings responsible for these conceptions were themselves the product of the experiences involved in a subconscious attempt to pass from a very low evolutionary, uncivilized stage to the higher civilized stage.

(3) During this transition, mental development had proceeded at a far greater rate proportionately than the physical, because physical development had already reached a high standard, and there was less possibility of development on that side (as development was then understood). Also, in the new way of life, there was relatively less demand on the "physical" and an increasing demand on the "mental."

(4) In civilization, with the increasing "mental" development, there has been a correspondingly gradual decrease in "physical" development in comparison to humanity's earlier periods when we roamed the plains and mountains in search of food.

(5) This was the beginning of an era when we interfered with the co-ordinated use and development of the psycho-physical organism.

From all this, we see, that up to a certain point, the more highly developed "physical" processes constituted the main guiding factor in human activity. Yet, in a comparatively short time, the relatively unused but more rapidly developing interdependent processes called "mind" were exalted to a higher place than the "body," only to be superseded by what those concerned called the "soul" —of which they knew even less than the little they knew about the "mind's" workings.

The very conception of a separation and class-distinction between "body, mind, and soul" indicates the presence of a more than
usually potent stimulus which could emanate only from a condition of overbalancing in some direction. As far as we can learn, the
poor body came into disgrace because of "the lusts of the flesh,"
themselves a natural result of malcoordination which, if we may
judge by the special laws which were formulated, would seem to
have shown up mainly in the sexual sphere. Else why should this
sphere have been particularly selected for condemnation, although
the satisfaction of the needs and desires of the reproductive system
is as essential as the satisfaction of the needs and desires of the
digestive system to the welfare of the individual and the race? The
desires and needs of these systems are normal and salutary as long
as moderation and not abuse is the rule. The evil of over-eating is
only equaled by that of over-drinking and surely the abuse of the
sexual act is intensified by one or the other, or both.

Indeed, "separation" in the human organism was an arbitrary
conception formed to fit in with certain stultifying premises which
human beings, probably in honesty and meekness of spirit, had laid
down and made a law unto themselves in striving to fulfill the
essential demands of the religious ideal.

This led naturally to that dreadful and debasing conception
which caused men and women actually to castigate the flesh, to
cut, as it were, a way to Heaven through the very fundamental of
their earthly being.

But the limit of the destruction wrought by this dissecting
process had not yet been reached. As education progressed, this
principle of a class-distinction within the organism grew and developed. The idea was cultivated that lack of knowledge in certain
specific spheres was the factor which must determine how clever
or ignorant a person was. A person might possess prodigious common sense, be a reasoning intelligent creature, but if he or she did
not happen to be versed in all the paraphernalia which made up the
curricula of the universities, schools, and colleges of their time,
they would be classified as ignorant.

Next followed the most stupid mistake made by subconsciously controlled people in education. It was a growing contempt for those who, despite their natural gifts, were thus classified as ignorant—especially for those whose work involved "physical" rather than "mental" demands. Together with this there was a wholly absurd and exaggerated admiration for those who worked in professions which were considered to demand almost exclusively "mental" activities.

(Note: This is only one of the many proofs we possess that the idea of a class-distinction lies at the very root of human make-up, and that despite all efforts that may be made by legislation or other external means to counter this idea, it will surely remain as a conviction until humankind has reached the reasoning stage of conscious guidance and control of the individual. Until this stage is reached, those ideals indicated by the words democracy, liberty, etc., are impossible of attainment.)

Need for Unity and Simplicity

Consideration of these facts makes us realize how far humanity had traveled from one of the original fundamentals of life, that is, unity, which must have existed from the beginning. It was a strange lack of reasoning that caused a false division in the indivisible psycho-physical unity of the organism.

A scientific friend recently asked me; "Why have we overlooked these important points for so long?" I referred him to the phrase which is now in such common use: "Life has become so complex." This is the crux of the whole matter and before we can unravel the horribly tangled skein of our present existence, we must come to a full *STOP*, and return to conscious, simple living, believing in the unity underlying all things, and acting in a practical way in accordance with the laws and principles involved.

In the midst of the worldwide tragedy we are witnessing now, a tragedy which seems still to be increasing since the Armistice [end of WWI—ed.], surely it is imperative that every individual must *stop*—in the fullest sense—and reconsider every particle of supposed knowledge, particularly "psychological" knowledge derived from general education, religious, political, moral, ethical, social, legal, and economic training, and ask the plain, straightforward question; "Why do I believe these things? By what process of reasoning did I arrive at these conclusions?"

If we are honest with ourselves in regard to our cherished ideas and ideals, the answer may at first prove a shock to us. The truth will be forced on us that much of our supposed knowledge is not real knowledge, and too often the boasted truth, a delusion. The majority of our cherished ideas and ideals are born out of impulse, or unbalanced emotion and prejudice, that is, ideas and ideals associated with a psycho-physical condition in the development of which unreliable sensory appreciation has played the leading part.

Need for Substituting in All Spheres the Principle of Prevention on a General Basis for Methods of "Cure" on a Specific Basis

Unreliable sensory appreciation has been, and still is, associated with a general deterioration in the health of humankind. Our conceptions and thoughts have been, and still are, conditioned by it, and lead to wrong conclusions and decisions in dealing with new problems. The best example of this is the choice of a specific "cure" on the "end-gaining" principle, namely "physical exercises." We estimated wrongly the relative value of the principles of prevention and "cure" and so neglected the "means," a principle necessary to all preventive procedure.

Each generation has made the same error and has built up a heavy burden for the succeeding one, in that the necessity for "cure" still continues to increase and will heap on the coming generations such a load as will be beyond the power of human endurance. Faulty sensory appreciation in the human beings of our time has caused them to become overbalanced in many directions and has deluded them into experimenting blindly in too many spheres. Disaster has followed such experiments in chemistry and death-dealing-machines, for instance, in the same way as it would follow the activities of children well supplied with powder and matches. The historian of a few centuries hence will be able to produce evidence of the psycho-physical state of the peoples of the twentieth century which will show that they have progressed little on the evolutionary plane beyond Stone Age man. That historian will also be able to show that during 1914–1918, human beings developed a new form of devilry and brutality that surpasses those of prehistoric humanity.

A psychological moment in human experience has undoubtedly arrived for a widespread consideration of the principle of prevention in its fullest application to human needs (in all "physical," "mental," and "spiritual" spheres). Comparing the proportion of human energy devoted to prevention and "cure," we find it, at present, to be about nine to one in favor of "cure." That this is so, after thousands of years of supposed civilization, gives food for reflection, because the idea of seeking a specific "cure" had its origin in the experiences of a lowly evolved human creature belonging to an earlier period of human development. It goes with a view of life which is narrow and limited, since it represents an attempt to gain an immediate "end" without consideration of larger issues.

We are, therefore, faced with the fact that too many of our cherished beliefs and attempts at reforms in all spheres are founded on the same instinctive procedures of our earlier ancestors, when they sought a "cure" in some herb or berry.

On the other hand, if prevention is the leading principle, we will not work for an immediate "end": its application, rather, is on a broad, constructive basis, without limits, humanly speaking and is the conception of a highly evolved type of human being.

Illustration 1

Let us consider what is known as the "liver cure":

A man has suffered certain symptoms for a year or more, is moved to see his doctor, and is told his liver is sluggish. He is given drugs and goes home with the conviction that all will now be well.

The plan is simple. If the symptoms recur he will swallow some more pills. This applies to a whole list of such "cures."

At this point I would beg my reader not to judge my standpoint until I have given my evidence. We, the people of the twentieth century, who consider that we can use our reasoning processes in far more spheres than our forebears, do not reason so well in connection with those problems on which our present and future well-being depends.

How does this person, then, reason about his sluggish liver? It is understandable that if he has an acute attack he should follow the doctor's orders to get clear, as he considers it, of a crisis. But why does the matter end here? The symptoms have been telling him for a long time that his liver is faulty, and he knows that he has been leading a sedentary life and overindulging in certain food and drink which are particularly gratifying to his not-too-reliable sensory appreciation (in this case particularly the sense of taste). This being so, one would expect him to show some intelligent recognition of the real situation. He does not, however, as he is set on a "cure" and continues to act on this "end-gaining" principle. He has never used his reasoning in connection with his psycho-physical well-being, never used any other principle than that of working for an immediate "end," because he is subconsciously controlled and in this connection his reasoning processes are in abeyance.

Interestingly, if one drug does not "cure" him, he will try another, and another, etc. This shows that in one narrow groove, at least, he is prepared to make changes, but he holds to the "cure" idea of the Stone Age by his confidence in drugs. In other words, he remains true to one of the most harmful habits which he has inherited as race instincts. He does not adopt the only principle a highly evolved human being could conceive of or tolerate, that is, the great comprehensive principle of *prevention*. He does not realize that something has gone wrong with the machinery of the whole organism.

For when a machine develops defects it cannot function at its maximum, and if the machine continues to be used, these defects become more pronounced and increase in number. In order to restore it to the maximum functioning, it is obvious that a knowledge of the motive, adjusting, guiding, and controlling principles of the mechanism is needed. In the case of the human mechanisms, a knowledge of the psycho-mechanical principles involved is necessary to their co-ordinated use, and this knowledge implies the possession of a sensory appreciation which is reliable.

If this sensory appreciation had continued to be reliable in civilization, how could defects in the organism have developed in a satisfactorily co-ordinated person? And if the sense registers are so unreliable and deceptive that a person can develop imperfections in the ordinary activities of life, what may be expected as a result of activities in remedial and other spheres, if he or she continues to be guided by the same sense registers that are deceiving them at every turn?

(Note: Many people may object to these arguments and refer to some defect which at some time they have removed, with or without aid. I am quite ready to admit this, but I assert that several other defects will have been cultivated in the process. I am prepared to prove this, if the objector will submit to examination. Incidentally, I may mention that these examinations are made while the subject remains fully dressed.)

The time is not far distant when these facts will be widely recognized. It will be realized that, in order to remove some defect, we will firstly have gradually to acquire a reliable sensory appreciation during a process of constructive conscious re-education.

Illustration 2

Let us consider another good illustration of a specific method—surgery. Before we do, however, I wish to make it clear that I fully appreciate the value of surgery in special spheres, and the good results obtained in these spheres. But it is possible that in the future surgeons could confer greater benefits on humankind than those they confer now, if they were to extend their field of operation and their outlook to include the wider plan of prevention.

Consider, for instance, the removal of the appendix or colon. If the surgeon concludes that an organ has deteriorated to the point of endangering the patient, then it will be removed. To this extent the sphere of surgery is confined within narrow limits.

Little consideration is given to the cause of the general interference with the functioning of the whole organism, an interference of which the *specific* deterioration in the appendix or colon is merely a symptom. No consideration is generally given to the fact that the operation, however skillfully performed, does not restore the reliable sensory appreciation necessary to the readjustment and co-ordination of the mechanism, so that vital activity will be restored and the dropped viscera caused to resume their normal, healthy position in the torso.

Therefore, the imperfect original functioning of the organism not only continues but is bound to become even more imperfect as time goes on. Surgery may then be needed again to give relief in a new direction.

Illustration 3

Let us consider psychoanalysis. I am prepared to demonstrate that this "cure" is based on the same specific "end-gaining" principles as the less modern methods which it is claimed by some to supersede. Take the person who suffers from some unreasoning fear. Between them, the teacher and the pupil unravel the knot and decide that the origin of the fear lies in some past event, or series of events, which unduly excited the fear reflexes and established a "phobia." Let us say a "cure" is made. What does this "cure" indicate? What fundamental change has taken place in the patient's psycho-physical condition?

Before answering these questions, we should take into consideration (as stated at the outset in this book) that all so-called mental activity is a process governed by our psycho-physical condition at the time a particular stimulus is received. This being so, it is obvious that the reason a person falls victim to some unreasoning fear is that their general psycho-physical condition at the time they receive the stimulus, to which fear is the reaction, is below a satisfactory standard.

(Note: It is common knowledge that a person is more subject to infections (colds, etc.) when "run down," that is, in a lowered psycho-physical condition.)

This patient must have been in a low state of psycho-physical functioning at the time the "phobia" was established. His kinesthetic sense was debauched and his sensory appreciation delusive. Psychoanalysis will not restore reliable sensory appreciation nor re-educate his psycho-physical mechanism on a general basis. The psycho-physical condition which permitted the establishment of the first phobia will permit another. All that is needed is the stimulus.

The method of psychoanalysis, therefore, like other methods of treatment on a subconscious basis, is an instance of an "end-gaining" attempt to effect the "cure" of a specific trouble by specific means, without consideration being given to the necessity of restoring a satisfactory standard of general psycho-physical functioning and of sensory appreciation.

Fundamental Defect in Our Plan of Civilization a Lack of Recognition of the Importance of the Principle of Prevention on a General Basis

It is the recognition in practice of the principle of prevention which makes possible our advance to higher and higher stages of evolution and opens up the greatest possibilities for human activities and accomplishment. I have insisted on this point because I wish to emphasize what, in my opinion, constitutes a fundamental defect in our plan of civilization, at least two thousands years old: in all attempts at improvement, human energy is spent on methods of specific cure instead of prevention. I have found that despite explaining this to pupils, I am still asked, "Have you ever 'cured' a case like mine?" I reply that I do not attempt to "cure" anyone. I merely look at the subject before me as a damaged machine, and in the light of my experience, ask myself if it is possible to restore a well co-ordinated condition of the psycho-physical organism as a whole.

(Note: Readers may ask, "Why, then, if you advocate the principle of prevention, do you work in a curative sphere?" The answer is simple. Firstly, the principle of prevention should be applied to children at a very early age. Secondly, up to now it has proved impossible to create a sufficient demand for fundamental psycho-physical re-education, to induce young people to study it with a view to teaching it professionally in the preventive sphere. This implies that their work must be confined to children.

The reader will see at once the difficulty that we face, that is, the inevitable law of supply and demand. Parents must first be convinced of the value of my technique before entrusting it to their children for the time necessary and in sufficient numbers to create a demand that will make it possible for young people to take up the work on a sound professional and financial basis. Up to now parents have said, "We will first come to you ourselves; then, if you are able to 'cure' us, we will consider the matter in relation to our children." It is in vain that I protest that I do not set out to "cure" anything. "You see," they reply, "for us to accept your work as the basis of our children's education means such a complete change in all our views and methods; it means practically beginning anew, and giving up so much that we have been taught is true up to now, that we cannot interfere with our children's education until we have proof of your work in ourselves."

Some of my scientific supporters are no less insistent on these points. Under these circumstances I am forced to work in a so-called curative sphere with adults, in the hope that they may help me in my efforts to gain a wide recognition of the necessity for the re-education on a general basis and for preventive measures for the children. Once we have created a demand amongst parents, the first part of the problem will be solved, for the supply will be there and will, in time, bring the right type of man or woman into the work. I am anxious and ready to devote the rest of my life, and the experience I have gained, relatively small though this may be, to preparing teachers to teach the children.

We need, therefore, to establish a school for the education of teachers. A number of people in England and America have been working with me to establish such a school. We are all aware of the harm we can do to the cause, if we attempt to do this too quickly, at the cost of training only those people who are able to bear the financial burden involved during the necessary years of training, irrespective of the standard to which the psycho-physical potentialities, which go to the making of a teacher, have been developed in their case: Such an attempt could end only in comparative failure, and in the long run do much to delay the wide acceptance of the principles involved.)

Instead, then, of trying to remove specific symptoms directly, I endeavor to bring about such re-adjustment of the organism *as a whole* that the symptoms in question disappear in the process, and are not likely to recur if the new conditions are maintained (principle of prevention).

In some pupils this is a long process, because it means a gradual building-up of new, satisfactory psycho-physical use based on a reasoning and not a blind acceptance of the principles involved. If, at the end of our talk, I consider that there is any doubt on the part of prospective pupils, I suggest that they read my book, and then, if they understand the principles, they should come to me for help. I beg them not to come simply because they believes I can "cure" them of something. I admit that anything will sometimes effect a "cure" as cure is generally understood; but the case of the exceptional "cure" by whatever means, medical or otherwise, cannot justify any reasoning person in attempting or promising a continuance of "cures" on these lines. All attempts to remove the causes of suffering which do not come within the scope of reasoned practical procedure must, with the broader view, be definitely abandoned. We should have passed that stage of ignorance and narrowness which permits the human being to entertain for a moment the idea of a miracle.

The miracle worker and the advocates of the "cure" methods have had free scope for over two thousand years, but despite this fact there has been a gradual increase in malconditions and therefore a correspondingly increasing need for a "cure."

I would even say that, in my opinion, the fact that humanity has not been guided by reasoning processes in connection with the problems of well-being is the reason for the tragedy of progress in civilization. The crisis of 1914 shows that we have released forces which we are unable to control, and by means of which millions of our fellow-beings have been swept from the earth. It would seem that humanity is simply preparing the way for its own extinction unless those energies, which in the past have been directed into harmful channels in the outside world, are in future directed and controlled by reasoning processes which have been employed primarily in the use of our psycho-physical organism.

This horrible recrudescence of barbarity is for the moment held in check. But, like a fire whose white-heated embers have been cooled by water on the outside—merely creating more heat inside—it will sooner or later burst once more into flame. Every ember representing an individual human being must be dealt with singly and separately, and if we are to prevent another fierce outbreak we must treat each ember in such a way that it will be as difficult to fire as it is to fire a stone.

Constructive conscious control will bring us nearer to that stage of evolutionary development where the masses, when thrown together, will no longer exhibit the inflammable traits associated with the herd instinct.

Our first efforts to rise above the depths from which many people today believe we will not be able to extricate ourselves, should be devoted to the establishment, in the individual, of a reliable sensory appreciation by means of conscious guidance. This is in order to prevent the recurrence of the disasters brought about in the past by people whose judgments, opinions, and policies have been based more on a deteriorated sense of feeling than on reasoning.

Think for a moment of the lack of reasoning associated, for instance, with a plan of life that allows the child, the adult of the future, to develop imperfections and defects, so that long before adolescence is reached, some curative method has to be adopted to remove these problems. With a reasoning plan of life, the principle of prevention would be fundamental in the child's education, *from the beginning*.

Attempts at education based on prevention will lead to much discussion and probably force me, by way of illustration, to set down descriptions of technical evolutions—a procedure which may seem to be an encouragement to people to cling to the "curative" and to neglect prevention. But I wish to free myself from responsibility for any such serious harm which invariably follows the attempt of the ordinary subconsciously controlled human being to follow written instructions for some exercise, etc., with the aim of eradicating a defect. I have already pointed out that even though a person may succeed by this means in eradicating some specific defect, he or she will be cultivating other defects; in what follows, I hope to make clear the reason for this generally unrecognized fact.

Because the fundamental shortcoming underlying all psycho-physical defects is delusive sensory appreciation, until satisfactory sensory appreciation is restored, *all exercises are a positive danger*. Reliable sensory appreciation is, therefore, essential and we will proceed to consider its part in any reasoned and satisfactory plan of education.

The rest of this volume, then, is devoted to an examination of the part played by sensory appreciation in education, taking this word in its broadest sense.

PART 2

SENSORY APPRECIATION IN ITS RELATION TO LEARNING AND LEARNING TO DO

Chapter 1

EDUCATION AND RE-EDUCATION

At no time in our history has the same general interest been shown in education (in its widest sense) as is manifested in the present day. The experiences of the War and the worldwide unrest which followed it have caused all thinking people to ask themselves searching questions about the validity of long-cherished beliefs in every sphere, and especially that of education. Articles about defects in our educational methods appear regularly in newspapers, and all kinds of new methods are being advocated. The state of confusion in the outside world is equally apparent in the educational world.

This confusion experienced in the practical application of educational theories is also to be found in our assessment of any particular system. This is because the merits or demerits of that system remain within the doubtful range of individual opinion, too often formed subconsciously, and based primarily on results.

I will try to make plain what, in my opinion, constitutes the fundamental cause of this confusion. I begin by first drawing attention to a well-known fact which is usually disregarded in all forms of education. This fact is that, whenever we wish to convey a new idea to someone—that is, to teach someone something—the person wishing to learn this new thing must first form a conception of what is indicated by the written or spoken words. His or her practical use of the new idea will be conditioned by this conception. This applies also when the individual tries to teach himself something. In acquiring knowledge, therefore, especially psychophysical knowledge, the person's conception is all-important: it is the construction which the learner places on what he hears or reads which determines the course of his actions and opinions.

Yet the ordinary teacher acts, and ordinary teaching methods are based, on the assumption that the pupil's conception of a new idea is identical to that of the teacher. Children frequently suffer disappointment and failure in their studies because they do not fully understand what is required of them. Every day in life, misunderstandings occur in trivial as well as in very important matters. The great majority of these misunderstandings occur because of some impeding factor which interferes with the process of reasoning. This process of reasoning is inseparable from what we call "understanding" or "mental conception."

The significance of the fact that a person's attempt to learn a new idea is conditioned by his or her conception, however, cannot be fully realized until we connect it with the further fact that this conception, in its turn, is conditioned by the standard of the individual's psycho-physical functioning. And, note again, that psycho-physical functioning depends on the standard of his sensory appreciation. In short, *the accuracy of the individual conception depends on the standard of psycho-physical functioning and of sensory appreciation.* Our total disregard of this fundamental fact is, in my opinion, the root of all the confusion in education and in every area of practical life.

To arrive at sound conclusions concerning the fundamentals on which education should be based, we must first consider the standard of psycho-physical functioning of the person who is to be educated, both today and in, what we hope will be, a progressive future. Unfortunately, a satisfactory standard of psycho-physical functioning has not been considered an essential in our schemes of education. We have depended mainly on subconscious guidance and control in our attempts to make "mental" progress. Modern educational methods are as lacking in this regard as the old ones.

Teachers and originators of modern systems are still trying to help individuals to progress towards a higher state of "physical" and "mental" development, while leaving them dependent on subconscious experiences for guidance and control. There is no consideration and no understanding of the harm done through attempts to obey instructions made by teachers who are themselves guided by unreliable and delusive sensory appreciation.

If a teaching technique is to be satisfactory, then it must meet the needs of human beings who are already saddled with varying and more or less serious defects in the employment of the mechanism. Let us outline some of these defects and the difficulties they present for both teacher and pupil in connection with children's activities at school.

The idea that a child should go to school is too often a preconceived idea with parents and not a reasoned conviction. The child is simply to be educated, which means to most people that he or she is to acquire knowledge and to be put "right" in matters where judged to be "wrong." All parents tend to have fixed ideas regarding present and future needs of the child, and choose a school in accordance with their ideas.

(Note: In a properly constituted civilization based on conscious control, parents would be trained to know their child's needs and to know how to satisfy them.)

Parents also have very definite ideas concerning what should be done in educating the child although they have no experience that would justify them holding these fixed opinions. Further, it occurs to very few of them to consider whether the child's fear reflexes will be harmfully excited by constant pressure from the teacher to always try to "be right."

(Note: The idea of "right" is almost always associated with *product or result,* not with *method* of operation. The instructions the child receives, such as, to "sit up straight," "speak out," "take a deep breath," "see how quietly you can walk," etc., are all specific "end-gaining" instructions which rarely include the "means" of carrying them out which could ensure satisfactory use of the psycho-physical mechanism.)

Children are made to feel that it is almost a disgrace to be wrong. Teachers do not know how to prevent even the very worst use in the child while standing or sitting at a desk pondering over a lesson. Cramming and other means adopted in learning cultivate harmful psycho-physical conditions—one result being recognized in a loss of memory, which in our time has become so serious that it has paved the way for educated people to be exploited by various "memory systems."

(Note: These systems are based on "specific" principles instead of satisfactory "psycho-physical" development. For example, it is well known that a sluggish liver adversely affects the functioning of the "mental" powers, that the person's reasoning powers are interfered with, and a temporary comparative loss of memory may occur. This fact underlines the interdependence of "mental" and "physical" activity. If the vital functioning of the "physical" organs is inadequate, the organism gradually becomes poisoned and the "mental" machinery gradually becomes less and less efficient. In such a case it is very difficult to understand in what mysterious way the ordinary memory system can enable one to remedy the "physical" disorders indicated, and if it does not, a successful result is highly improbable. See chapter on "Memory and Feeling.")

Undue excitement of the fear reflexes in the daily school work has a very serious effect on the breathing, which is so closely linked up with the emotions. In addition, if we consider the detrimental effect on the breathing and emotions in the defective use of the organism during study at desks and in school chairs, or during the assumption of any ordinary posture, we are faced with a problem which no scheme on a subconscious basis will solve. (As Byron wrote: "Breathless as we stand when feeling most.") These are tremendous impeding factors in the child's activities.

In attempting to improve handwriting, for instance, new faults will be developed in the general use of the psycho-physical mechanisms, and established defects will tend to become more pronounced. Knowledge acquired in this way is gained at the cost of losing co-ordinated control, particularly with the use of those psycho-physical mechanisms on which respiratory control depends. With these conditions present, the child lacks the psycho-physical equipment essential to the best efforts in learning something. The gradual lowering of the respiratory and other vital processes during study is undoubtedly one of the impeding factors which make for the dreamy condition—often amounting almost to stupor—into which people of the student and orthodox "thinking class" drift.

I admit that there is a steadily growing minority of parents who want more for their children than reading, writing and arithmetic, who want their children to have a "complete and all-round development." In certain areas of education there have been changes and some attempts have been made to counter supposed defects. Unfortunately, these attempts are too often merely a reaction from one extreme to another. They fail because they are based on a principle of specific, not general, development. The child is not treated as a *whole* organism, and it is not recognized that the child of today does not start life with the standard of co-coordination and sensory appreciation enjoyed by the child of, say, 200 years ago. Today's psycho-physical mechanisms are not nearly as reliable; by the time the ordinary child reaches school age, certain wrong uses of the organism have already become established, constituting a serious condition which baffles the most thoughtful teachers. As one teacher wrote, "No one who observes carefully the predominant characteristics of the present generation can fail to note:

(1) Alarming imperfections of the physique, i.e., defects of spine, wrong posture, lack of muscular co-ordination, depressed stature, etc.

(2) Limitations in the mental field, that is, domination by a fixed idea, inability to apprehend and to respect other points of view, failure to grasp the essentials of freedom, etc."

All this is symptomatic of some underlying cause.

The head of an important preparatory school consulted me in the hope of solving what she considered *the problem* of the school. Although all the most recent educational methods, satisfactory environmental conditions, outdoor activity, and "free-expression" had been adopted at the school, the problem remained, while the urgency for its solution became more and more apparent. She admitted that until she had read *Man's Supreme Inheritance* she could not understand why the active outdoor life did not eradicate the physical shortcomings in the children causing concern. But of what avail are all these things if the child is actually allowed to use him or herself during their activities in a way that is harmful, and interferes so much with the respiratory processes that these are used to the minimum rather than maximum capacity? Teachers agree that the proper working of these processes is the most vital element in the child's development.

The almost universal call from parents and teachers for physical exercises, posture training, breathing exercises, etc., in schools is an admission of a great need. But these methods will not give the necessary help. A child's harmful habits acquired during study cannot be remedied by physical exercises or any other of the methods mentioned above.

The problem is further complicated by the fact that there is a continual increase in the educational demands made on the child—unavoidably, it is supposed, in the present stage of civilization. This causes an increase in malcoordination in the same ratio as the difficulties to be overcome in any attempt to eradicate defects. Also, the degree of difficulty which the child will encounter in lessons will be in accord with the degree of imperfect general functioning. To be successful the child has then to devote more and more time to these subjects, so that increasing demands are being made on him or her—involving longer hours of work, increased effort, and the increasing complications these imply. How can the psycho-physical mechanisms of children meet these demands satisfactorily when they are functioning so much nearer to their minimum than to their maximum possibilities? And what will happen if educational demands continue to increase, while the children's psycho-physical possibilities continue to decrease—as they surely will, unless these defects are eradicated and a process of genuine development on a plane of conscious control is set in motion?

If teachers attempt to remedy a *specific* defect in a malcoordinated child (say for instance in handwriting), they must take into account the standard of general psycho-physical functioning in the child, otherwise new faults will develop and old ones will be reinforced.

We cannot expect the best results in the acquisition of knowledge if psycho-physical functioning is more or less inadequate. The child's early efforts to learn any simple subject are based on *specifics,* that is, on "end-gaining" principles of trying to do specific things "right." Long before adolescence is reached, this "end-gaining" procedure will have become established. This will be associated with a bad psycho-physical attitude towards accepting new ideas and new experiences, and too often with a serious deterioration in memory. When these defects are present, they constitute two impeding factors which could account for the general lack in the majority of adults to link up knowledge. Knowledge is of little use in itself; it is the linking up of what we know with that which comes to us daily in the shape of new ideas and new experiences which is of value, and this ability to link up is inseparable from the processes concerned with remembering. In other words, the value of knowledge lies in our power to make use of it in association with the greater knowledge which should come to us as we increase in years of experience, and as we substitute reasoning for instinct and for what Professor Dewey calls "emotional gusts."

Education, therefore, must first secure for the child the highest possible standard of psycho-physical functioning. In this way children will make a fair start, and will continue to improve the conditions involved in their efforts as pupils in all other activities.

The plan of education which I advocate is a comprehensive one which not only meets the needs of the human being at this stage of evolution, but will also meet future needs as we pass from subconscious guidance to a higher and higher state of civilization. The test of our advance in this connection demands a consideration of:

(1) the plane of consciousness reached in our recognition of incorrect psycho-physical use within the organism, and in our use of that organism in everyday life;

(2) the standard of our ability to accept readily, new and expanding ideas, when we have become convinced of their value and their superiority to old, long-cherished ideas, together with a keen desire for new experiences and for a standard of use which will enable us to profit by these experiences;

(3) the standard of our ability to adapt to the rapid changes in civilization with benefit, not detriment, to our psycho-physical self.

(4) the standard of our ability to check our fear of giving up our job and boldly to make the necessary change should we find that the fundamental principles concerned are defective; and/or to make adjustments essential to the acceptance and assimilation of new and approved knowledge while going on with one's job.

The consideration of principles in connection with any plan of education leads naturally to the consideration of the *means* of any technique, to the *how* of carrying the principles out.

All teaching methods on a subconscious basis are formed on the principle that if the pupil suffers from some defect, he or she must at once *do something* (with the help of the teacher) to eradicate it. The teacher believes in this system for dealing with defects. It is his or her business to teach the pupil to do something to eradicate defects. The "doing" in this connection means to the pupil simply *the performance of a series of physical movements to be carried out in accordance with the pupil's conception of the teacher's instructions.* The fact that pupils fail in the great majority of cases may disturb the teacher, but it does not lessen his or her faith in the methods. They may point to some successes, but teachers are not aware enough to see that these successes are merely *specific,* and that in eradicating the particular defect the pupil has been allowed to cultivate several others more harmful than the original, and of which teacher and pupil alike remain ignorant.

On the other hand, a teaching procedure using constructive conscious control is based on the opposite principle: that people whose sensory appreciation is deceptive cannot expect to remedy their condition by relying on the same deceptive feeling in their efforts to re-educate themselves or to put right something they know to be wrong in the organism. In the attempt to perform any act, habit and inherited and cultivated instincts remain the dominating factor.

The significance of this in relation to education can be understood fully if we follow the argument a step further. If a teacher asks a boy who is experiencing difficulty in carrying out an activity to *do anything by himself* in order to overcome the difficulty or eradicate defects, *the only guidance the child has to rely on in doing anything to carry out the teacher's instruction is the very same delusive subconscious guidance (unreliable sensory appreciation) that was the cause of the defects developing and becoming established in the first place:* This applies with even greater force when applied to adults. All psycho-physical defects are symptoms of malcoordination and maladjustment hand in hand with faulty sensory appreciation. Any attempt to eradicate defects using the same faulty sensory appreciation as a guide merely exaggerates them and results in undue development of the fear reflexes.

A technique to meet this difficulty is required, a technique that involves correct manipulation on the part of the teacher in order to give the pupil correct experiences in sensory appreciation, experiences of re-education, readjustment, and co-ordination. Further, in order to give these satisfactory sensory experiences, the teacher must him or herself be in possession of a reliable sensory mechanism and have gained the experience in re-education and co-ordination that is required for a satisfactory readjustment of the organism.

But it must be clearly understood that the correct sensory experiences cannot be described in writing or by the spoken word. As a friend of mine, a well-known scientific man, replied to a question in this connection: "We cannot write a kinesthesia, any more than we can write the sense of sound. We can only write the symbols of sound, notes of music, for instance."

It is necessary to emphasize this point, as it is one that is constantly overlooked. Many people have said to me, with a friendly knowing look: "That book of yours, *Man's Supreme Inheritance*, is quite a clever piece of work: you give us enough to make us interested in your theory and just lead us to the point where we realize we must go to you for lessons!" Many times I have demonstrated to a pupil that he needs re-education because of his lack of reliable sensory appreciation, that he is guiding himself by deceptive "feeling," and often the reply has been: "Please give me some exercise that I can practice at home." I have emphasized in my book the point that manipulation is necessary for developing and establishing reliable sensory appreciation; but I am still criticized for "keeping things back" because I do not give instructions and exercises for the pupil to *do* at home, *by themselves*. I point out that I will not be guilty of adding to the mass of literature on the subject of exercises, or take the grave responsibility for the harmful consequences of such exercises, carried out according to written instructions by people whose sensory appreciation is unreliable and often positively delusive. My technique has been developed throughout from the premise that, if something is wrong with us, it is because we have been guided by unreliable sensory appreciation, leading to wrong sensory experiences, resulting in misdirected activities.

These misdirected activities manifest themselves in our use in all the general activities of life, and in many varying ways according to our individual idiosyncrasies. They are influenced by and associated with our incorrect conceptions, our imperfect sensory appreciation, our unduly excited fear reflexes and uncontrolled emotions and prejudices, and our imperfectly adjusted mechanisms. As these psycho-physical defects develop, they create an attitude in the conduct of life in general which must be considered perverted. And because these misdirected activities are so closely connected with this perverted attitude, they present a difficult problem to both teacher and pupil in any attempt to convey or acquire knowledge—particularly in regard to the satisfactory use of the psycho-physical mechanisms. I shall, therefore, now go on to consider this problem in its relation to incorrect conception.

Chapter 2

INCORRECT CONCEPTION

The first step is to convince the pupil that his or her present misdirected activities are the result of incorrect conception and imperfect sensory appreciation (feeling).

However, the pupil will usually not be convinced of this by discussion and argument alone. Pupils will often say that they see the argument, and from their standpoint this may be true. But, in my experience, the only way to really convince pupils that their sense of feeling is misleading them when they make a movement is by *demonstration on the pupil's own organism.* A mirror should be used so that the pupil can see the difference.

The next point of importance is to impress on the pupil the importance of listening carefully to the teacher's words and to be quite clear as to their intended meaning, *before the pupil attempts to act on them.* This may seem a truism, but it is a rock on which even a highly experienced teacher may make shipwreck, because the pupil's conception of what the teacher is trying to convey by words *will be in accordance with the pupil's psycho-physical make-up.* In this sense, it may truly be said that a person hears only what he or she wants to hear.

If a person has fixed ideas, these must inevitably limit their capacity for "listening carefully." Therefore the teacher must give due consideration to the pupil's fixed conceptions; otherwise these will greatly complicate the problem. Certain of these fixed ideas are encountered in the case of almost every pupil, for example, as to what constitutes the right and wrong method of going to work as a pupil; fixed ideas about the necessity for concentration; a fixed belief that if a pupil is corrected, he or she should be taught *to do something in order to correct it, instead of being taught, as a first principle, how to prevent (inhibition) the wrong thing from being done.*

An experienced teacher can see, by the expression in the use of the pupil's eyes, the degree of influence of such conceptions. At each step in the training, the teacher should take preventive measures to counteract this influence. It is absurd to try to teach a person who is in an agitated or anxious condition. We must have a calm condition which is characteristic of a person whose reasoning processes are operative.

A teaching experience of twenty-five years has given me a very real knowledge of the psycho-physical difficulties which stand in the way of many adults who need re-education and co-ordination. I have no hesitation in saying that fixed ideas and conceptions form the major part of their difficulties.

Let us consider some examples from my teaching experience, because they are so widespread and have such harmful effects on life in general. I will begin with the habit which has become established in most people trained on a subconscious basis, one referred to earlier, *that of trying to correct one defect by doing something else.*

Illustration 1

"Doing It Right"

In the first lesson, the teacher explains that the pupil has certain psycho-physical peculiarities which the teacher proposes to attempt to eradicate, and then explains the *means* of doing so.

The pupil inevitably and unavoidably forms his or her own conception of what this means. Unless the pupil is a very unusual person, he will have come to a decision based on his preconceived ideas. She will think that she will be required *to do something* (as she understands "doing") *and do it right* (as she understands "doing it right"). It is probable that all their former teachers have instilled the habit of trying to get something right whenever it is wrong. They will also have been told that if they are conscientious, they will always try to be right, not wrong. Further, this desire to "be right" will have become an obsession in which, as in many other matters, his or her conscience must be satisfied.

(Note: Consideration of this will force us to admit that a person's insistence on satisfying conscience is merely an attempt to unload responsibility. The person is aware of certain orthodox ways of dealing with his difficulties, but they generally fail. Still they argue that if they try them and they fail, at least they have done their best. In other words, they try to satisfy their conscience, not their reasoning intelligence. They use this way of going about things because it is the easy way. If they stopped to reason the thing out, and looked at the experience gained from previous failure, they would realize that they would have to discard these orthodox methods and seek new ones. This would be the difficult way. It would mean a careful dissection of their psycho-physical peculiarities, defects, prejudices, and sensory excesses. These are to them just as much a manifestation of his their malconditions as is the diseased liver for the drunkard. To give his liver a chance, the drunkard would have to give up drinking, but he has not the control to do this. So it is with the pupil in our illustration. She knows that certain psycho-physical habits are responsible for her condition, but these habits have become a part of her; they appeal to her perverted sense of feeling, and so she will not make the effort to give them up.)

As soon as the teacher observes that the pupil is setting out to do something he thinks "right" in accordance with his fixed ideas, he must show the pupil that by "doing something" himself, he is relying on his own *judgment, but that his judgment cannot be sound in this respect, because it is based on previous incorrect sensory experiences.* The teacher, therefore, asks the pupil to stop relying on his own judgment in these matters, and, instead, to listen to the new instructions, and allow the teacher, by means of manipulation, to give him the new, correct sensory experiences.

The idea of ceasing to do the wrong thing, (as a preliminary measure in re-education) does not at first, appeal to the average pupil, who, in most cases, goes on trying to be "right."

The main reason for this, as I have pointed out, is that in our conception of how to employ the different parts of our mechanisms, we are guided almost entirely by an unreliable sense of feeling. We get into the habit of performing a certain act in a certain way and this makes it feel "right." *The act and the particular feeling associated with it become one in our recognition.* If something causes us to change our conception, however, about the manner of performing the act, and if we adopt a new method in accordance with this changed conception, we will experience a *new feeling* which we do not recognize as "right." We then realize that what we have recognized as being "right" has been wrong all the time.

For example, the pupil is asked to bend his knees. The pupil, thinking only of what the teacher asks him, (the "end"), and wishing to do it right, (as he understands "doing it right"), bends them as he has always done—with too much tension and pressure, interfering with his equilibrium, shortening his spine, and stiffening his neck. Thus he achieves his end, the bending of the knees, but at the cost of undue strain and disadvantage to the organism. Of course, the pupil is not conscious of all this. He has probably never thought out *how* he has performed such acts as "bending the knees"; and although he knows in a general way that something is wrong with him, he has never associated this "something wrong" with anything that *he has been doing himself.* Therefore, bending his knees in his usual manner satisfies him, *it feels right to him.*

Suppose that the teacher manages to get the pupil to bend his knees to the best advantage in the general use of his mechanisms. (Details in the following chapters.) For the pupil, the act of bending the knees then *becomes a new act, bringing with it a new feeling,* but as it is not what he is accustomed to, it will *feel wrong.*

The pupil now has a choice whenever he wishes to bend his knees: the old way or the new way, "feeling right" or "feeling wrong." As a little girl said when this was explained to her: "Oh, I see! If I feel at all, I must feel wrong. If I don't feel wrong, I mustn't feel." Unfortunately, the average adult pupil, unlike the little girl, does not "see," or, if he does, cannot or will not act accordingly. In fact, the adult, as a rule, does not like a new feeling, and in some cases is positively *afraid* of it. A new "feeling" gives him or her a sense of insecurity. This sense of insecurity is particularly marked in connection with the maintaining of equilibrium in standing, walking, etc., in the new way, with the newly acquired feeling.

(Note: Incidentally, when people develop phobias about crossing streets, being alone in a room, traveling by train or plane, crossing bridges or open spaces, are unduly alarmed by sudden noises, etc., there is already a serious condition of unsatisfactory psycho-physical equilibrium, which accounts for the susceptibility to the particular stimulus responsible for the "phobia.")

And so it happens that, when a pupil is faced with the alternative of using his mechanisms badly and "feeling right" or of using them well and "feeling wrong," he is likely to "lose his head" and, instead of stopping to consider (that is, inhibit), fall back on "feeling right."

In such cases as the one described, the pupil's fixed ideas about "right" or "wrong" will produce a deadlock. For how can new and correct experiences be given to a pupil, who, in all the movements he makes, is working subconsciously to reproduce certain feelings that he has grown used to and likes? The situation is one that no teacher, however expert, can deal with satisfactorily until the pupil learns to stop trying to get things right, stops, that is, working blindly for his ends. He must give thought, instead, to the *means* of achieving his ends.

Illustration 2

Doing Things "My Way"

Another unreasoned conception common amongst pupils is their fixed ideas about *what they can and cannot do.*

Their judgment is based on their previous misleading experiences; but they are not ready to change their ideas, even when the teacher has given them practical proof that their judgment on these points cannot be relied on. It would seem reasonable that any pupil who seeks lessons from a teacher because he or she thinks the teacher can help them would take the teacher's word for it regarding what they are capable of doing or not. But too often the opposite is the case, because if the teacher asks pupils to do something which they are convinced they cannot do, then pupils will immediately falter. They may not openly refuse to carry out the new instructions, but they will make a "mental reservation" when they receive them. This is because they subconsciously believe they know more than the teacher about what they can or cannot do. So, pupils start carrying out the instructions on a plan of their own, that is in what he or she calls "my way." They can be so intent on this plan that the new instructions do not reach their consciousness—that is, do not make the necessary impression on them which would enable them to carry out the instructions satisfactorily, or even to remember them accurately.

Curiously, a pupil's confidence in "my way" is in no way disturbed by the fact that "my way" has been so unsuccessful in the past, even when the teacher shows that this "my way" *is essentially wrong for the pupil's purpose.* In fact, what the pupil considers a "difficulty" is not a difficulty in itself, but simply the result of "his or her way" of going to work.

Further, the teacher will point out that any reason the pupil may have had in the past for clinging to "his way" is no longer existent, because the presence of a teacher who can give practical help changes the situation. All the pupil has to do is to stop trying to overcome her difficulty "her way" and instead to follow the new instructions.

This is not an unreasonable proposition, if we have once decided that the teacher should be trusted to know more than the pupil about this particular matter. However, in general people are not attracted to this form of reasoning when faced with a "difficulty."

So the pupil continues to *try and do it his way,* although the teacher demonstrates over and over again that he cannot do what he is *trying* to do unless he changes the *means* of doing it.

If the pupil can adopt the new means given to him *he will be able to do quite easily the thing he has always believed he cannot do.* However, if he cannot, and goes on trying to be right "his way," he finds that after a time he is worrying, because he is not making progress. In other words, "his way" is not working. Could anything be more unreasonable?

Suppose a man sets out to reach a certain destination and comes to a fork in the road. Not knowing the way, he takes the wrong road of the two and gets lost. He asks someone he meets and is told to go back to the fork and take the other road. What would we think if we heard that he had gone back to the fork, but had there decided that he knew better than his adviser, and again taken his old road? And this not only once, but over and over again, getting lost, and still more, actually worrying about the fact that he is lost?

The reader is probably thinking that he or she would not be guilty of *not really attempting to do* that which he or she knows they *can* do, or of *not ceasing to try to do* that which the experience of years has proved to be *the impossible* in their particular case. Yet this is so with more or less every pupil, even those considered the most intelligent, the most highly educated, the most scientifically trained. *This strengthens my conviction that the principles underlying present methods of education are erroneous. Indeed, these methods have tended actually to cultivate this defect.* "Defect" is a word that is inadequate to express what really amounts to the loss of one half of our original psycho-physical endowment by the gradually decreasing use of the invaluable process called inhibition. Those who are responsible for these educational methods have not realized the importance of holding the balance true, in every sphere of life, between the desire to do (volition) and the ability to check that desire (inhibition).

The words "volition" and "inhibition" are in constant use in this book, and the way they are used must be clearly understood. Volition stands for the act of *responding* to stimuli to psycho-physical action (doing); inhibition stands for the act of *refusing to respond* to stimuli to psycho-physical action (non-doing). In other words, volition is used to name *what we intend to do,* and inhibition to name *what we refuse to do,* what we wish to *prevent.*

The problem of whether volition and inhibition are different manifestations of the same force, or even what this force is, does not need to concern us here. I believe that, before we acquire accurate knowledge about the nature of inhibition, we may possibly have solved volition—by means of that consciously acquired knowledge which is coming to us through the practical understanding of our psycho-sensory potentialities, on which a higher and higher standard of human psycho-physical functioning depends.

In the sense, then, implied by a process concerned with enabling one to stop, concerned not with "ends" —however good in themselves—but with the "means" of bringing these "ends" about, I maintain that there is a lack of inhibition in all spheres of life. The lack of inhibitory development in the use of the mechanism in the activities of everyday life is particularly fraught with danger, however, because this lack tends to produce a state of unbalanced psycho-physical functioning in the whole organism. Indeed, all our methods of educational training make for rigidity rather than mobility. Small wonder, then, that adults in whom such psycho-physical conditions have become established during childhood, show an almost total lack of the most ordinary common sense in

their activities in conjunction with unreliable sensory appreciation.

Illustration 3

Not Seeing Ourselves As Others See Us

Perhaps the most striking instance of human delusion is found in
our attitude towards our own psycho-physical defects, peculiarities, etc., on the one hand, and our merits and natural gifts on the
other. "To thine own self be true" is an inspiring incentive when
the human being's co-ordinated psycho-physical development has
reached a point where that self cannot be duped by its sensations.

Consider someone who stutters. He has certain beliefs about
the things he thinks of as "right" or "wrong" in himself concerning
speaking in everyday life. One of my pupils, a bad stutterer, learned
in a short space of time to speak without stuttering as long as he
spoke slowly. I asked him to speak in this new way during conver-
sations throughout his whole day. The pupil at once became
agitated, thus disturbing his new and developing control, and
relapsed into his old way of stuttering, and said; "Oh, I couldn't
do that, everyone would notice me!"

If we analyze the condition of a person who can seriously make
a remark like this quite sincerely, we will see that his agitation
caused him to revert to his old malcoordinated condition, a condition in which he had been used to hypnotize himself about the
facts of his shortcomings and peculiarities. We could say that he
was so used to his stuttering that he no longer cared what anyone
else thought about it, or that he had decided to ignore the disagreeable fact that he stuttered, and had deluded himself into
thinking that nobody else noticed his contortions.

(Note: This is the opposite delusion to that of the person who
becomes self-conscious about a comparatively unnoticeable
peculiarity and thinks that everywhere he goes people are
looking at him. This person does not realize that this defect
is so slight that nobody else notices it.)

The stutterer, then, has reached a stage of defective sensory appreciation and self-hypnotic indulgence that has made his whole outlook topsy-turvy. He no longer sees things as they are. Therefore, he is able to persuade himself that the *normal condition would be conspicuous, while the abnormal one would pass unnoticed. In this he is relying on his perverted sense of feeling.* The point to stress here is that delusion and self-deception are more or less present in all people who are imperfectly co-ordinated and have unreliable sensory appreciation.

Illustration 4

"Out of Shape"

In connection with unreliable sensory appreciation and incorrect conceptions of what is "right" or "wrong," the following is a significant example.

A little girl was brought to me. She had been unable to walk properly for years. After I had worked on her for a little while and had straightened out some twists and distortions in her body, she turned to her mother and said: "Oh, Mummy, he's pulled me *out of shape*."

This shows that the little girl's sensory apparatus told her that her "out-of-shape" condition was "in-shape." Imagine, then, what would be the result of her trying to get anything "right," by doing something herself in practicing remedial exercises recommended by a teacher. Small wonder that all attempts to teach her had failed.

Think also of the psycho-physical condition of this child when she reached adolescence, if the orthodox methods of teaching her had continued. Her faulty sensory awareness caused incorrect conceptions of herself, resulting in harmful experiences which were a positive danger to her future development. Unless in such cases a child is re-educated on a basis of conscious control, it cannot acquire a reliable sensory appreciation and all its efforts in the activities of life will be in accordance with this standard of functioning.

The point that comes out clearly in all these illustrations is *that conceptions which are mainly influenced by unreliable sensory appreciation, which acts and reacts subconsciously and harmfully on the processes involved, are incorrect conceptions, and that in these cases, unreliable sensory appreciation goes hand in hand with incorrect and deceptive experiences in the psycho-physical functioning.* Our judgment is based on experience, so, where this experience is incorrect and deceptive, the resulting judgment will be misleading and out of touch with reality. *We have to recognize, therefore, that our sensory peculiarities are the foundations of what we think of as our opinions, and that nine out of ten of the opinions we form are the result of what we feel, rather than what we think.*

(Note: It is reasonable to conclude that it is because the opinions of most people are based on feeling rather than reasoning that there are so many varied and conflicting opinions about some simple single point, or serious subject. It is positively alarming that reasoning plays so small a part in most of the opinions we hold in things that matter. This is why we find ourselves in such a fearful muddle after two thousand years of struggle towards a better standard of psycho-physical functioning, a struggle which it was hoped would bring in an era of goodwill, universal unity, tolerance, and mutual understanding.)

Our emotional defects are also linked up with our sensory peculiarities, so that, given the slightest disturbance in these directions, we must be temporarily thrown into a danger zone where serious and uncontrolled psycho-physical conditions prevail.

(Note: It only needs a certain number of repetitions of such harmful experiences to produce one or other of the different phases which border on insanity. Many phases of this development of temporary insanity are accompanied by violent physical manifestations.)

We can now see how far this line of thought has brought us. The fact that constantly emerges is *that our approach to life*

*generally, our activities, beliefs, emotions, opinions, and judg-
ments in whatever sphere are conditioned by the preceding conceptions, which are associated with the individual use of the
psycho-physical mechanisms and conditioned by the standard of
reliability of our individual sensory appreciation.*

This is the great fact which must be realized by our leaders in
educational, religious, moral, social, political, and all other spheres
of human activities before there can be any "uplifting" of the human being out of the present chaotic conditions. We all think
and act (except when forced to do otherwise) in accordance with
the peculiarities of our particular psycho-physical make-up. We
read a particular newspaper each morning because the policy of
that paper is the one we believe in; we cultivate friendships with
people who think as we think, and ignore, or are antagonized by,
those who do not; the preacher attracts to church only those who
want to go to church; we start to read a book, but when we reach
a point with which we disagree, our faulty kinesthesia cannot
control the impulses which, when set in motion, put us out of
touch with our reasoning. Yet, in spite of all this, books are written,
lectures given, sermons preached, and speeches made in the belief
that ideas given out in this way can be satisfactorily assimilated by
listeners or readers, and that good ideas may thus be passed on for
the uplifting of mankind.

Here we have a great delusion, because our ability to assimilate
unfamiliar ideas, or to overcome our prejudices, depends on our
individual conception of such ideas and beliefs, and this conception is conditioned by the standard of individual psycho-physical
co-ordination and of reliability of sensory appreciation. Had this
fact not been overlooked, writers, lecturers, preachers, etc., would
long since have shown some practical interest in the *means* by
which their hearers and readers could reach such a standard of
psycho-physical functioning that they would be able to assimilate
satisfactorily new ideas and teachings. For how, I ask, can people
who have developed a condition of unreliable sensory appreciation (with all the associated incorrect experiences, beliefs, and

judgments) assimilate satisfactorily ideas that do not fit in with these experiences? Correct apprehension and reliable sensory appreciation go hand in hand. (As a friend, a doctor, wrote to me recently: "I am getting more and more convinced that people can learn only what they know.")

The mass is made up of individuals, and reliable sensory appreciation cannot be given on the mass teaching principle or by precept or exhortation. This can only be done by individual teaching and individual work. Further, people who are massed together are likely to be governed by "herd instinct," and we need to help humankind to evolve beyond that influence as soon as possible. To this end, we must have conscious and individual development.

Chapter 3

IMPERFECT SENSORY APPRECIATION

The problem, then, is to find the *means* of developing and *maintaining* reliable sensory awareness. In both education and re-education this must be brought about in every case by the reliance of the individual, not on subconscious, but on *conscious, reasoning* guidance and control.

The connection between psycho-physical defects and incorrect sensory guidance must be recognized by the teacher in the practical work of re-education. The recognition of this vital connection marks the point of departure between methods of teaching on a conscious and on a subconscious basis.

I will now outline the general scheme which I advocate for developing reliable sensory appreciation—first setting out the principles, and then giving illustrations showing the application of these principles to the practical work of co-ordination and re-education.

First, the teacher must recognize the almost alarming dominance of the pupil's psycho-physical processes by an incorrect sensory appreciation in attempting to do something. It is of primary importance that the teacher points this unreliable sensory appreciation out to the pupil, and then helps him or her to develop new and reliable sensory appreciation.

The procedure is as follows: The teacher expertly manipulates the pupil's mechanisms to give the pupil the new sensory experiences required for a satisfactory use, whilst at the same time asking the pupil to think the correct guiding directions which are the counterpart of the new sensory experiences.

This procedure constitutes the *means* by which the teacher makes it possible for the pupil to *prevent* (inhibition) the misdirected activities which are causing his or her imperfections. The inhibitory process must take first place and remain the primary factor in each and every new experience which is to be gained and become established during the development of reliable sensory appreciation on which a satisfactory standard of co-ordination depends.

From the beginning, the teacher carefully explains that the pupil's part in this scheme is very different from that which is usually assigned to pupils in other teaching methods. The teacher tells the pupil that, on receiving the directions, he or she must not attempt to carry them out. On the contrary, *they must inhibit the desire to do so in the case of each and every direction which is given to them.* They must instead think the directions while the teacher, at the same time, will make the required re-adjustments using manipulation and bring about the necessary co-ordinations. In other words, the teacher performs the movements for the pupil and gives him or her the new and reliable sensory appreciation, and the very best opportunity possible to connect the different guiding directions before putting them into practice. This linking-up of the directions is all-important, because it is the counterpart of that linking-up of the parts of the organism which constitutes what we call co-ordination. The aim of re-education on a general basis is to bring about at all times and for all purposes, not a series of correct positions or postures, *but a co-ordinated use of the mechanisms in general.*

The second point to be noted in this technique is that the directions given to the pupil are based on the principle of ceasing to work blindly for some "end," so that he or she can pay attention instead to the "means" of achieving such an end. We have already considered this principle in general, but I wish to stress once again that it is of the utmost importance. Pupils must be able to accept this principle and apply it to their work in re-education because they cannot overcome their old subconscious habits by any other method, and so build up consciously the new improved conditions they are anxious to bring about.

If we pause to consider this, we will see that if the pupil thinks of a certain "end" and pursues it directly, he will take the course of action that he is accustomed to taking (i.e., following his habitual procedure). If this procedure happens to be a bad one for the purpose, he only strengthens his incorrect experiences. If, on the other hand, the pupil *stops himself* from doing it in his usual way (inhibition), and replaces his habit by the new conscious means, he will have taken the first most important step towards the breaking-down of a habit, and towards that constructive, conscious, reasoning control which tends towards a mastery of the situation. This applies in every sphere of activity.

The teacher impresses on the pupil from the beginning that, as the essential preliminary to any successful work by the pupil, *he must refuse to work directly for his "end," and keep his attention entirely on the "means" of securing the "end."*

In the illustration which will shortly be given, it will be seen that it is left to the teacher's discretion whether, in some movement, the pupil will be told beforehand what the "end" is. In every case, the pupil is told that the "end" does not matter, because given:

(1) that the teacher knows the correct "means" of achieving the "end"

(2) that the pupil understands how to give repeated conscious directions relating to these "means"

(3) that manipulation by the teacher's expert hands gives the pupil the reliable sensory appreciation which should result from the directions,

it is then merely a matter of time before the desired "end" is reached. In other words, the pupil is asked to take care of the "means" and the "end" will take care of itself.

(Note: In this connection, the length of time taken in the process of re-education before the new experiences can become established has proved a stumbling block for some enquirers. But again, if we reason the matter out, we shall see that the ability to break long-established habits depends on certain natural qualities in the pupil, especially on the standard of acuteness of sense perceptions and on the development of the ability to inhibit.)

In this way, all responsibility for the final result is taken off the pupil. He has no "end" to work for, nothing to get right. He is asked, when he receives a guiding order, to *listen and wait*; to wait, because only by waiting can he prevent himself from relapsing into his subconscious habits, and to listen, so that he learns to remember gradually and connect up the directions which are the counterpart of the "means" which the teacher is using to bring about the desired "end." In other words, he is asked to adopt consciously a principle of prevention as the basis of his practical work, and in every other way to leave the teacher a free hand.

Pupils who are willing to remain quietly giving directions to themselves at the prompting of the teacher, leaving to the teacher the responsibility of enabling them to bring about the desired results, are relieved of strain and anxiety and are able to gain the new and correct experiences with a gradually increasing sense of power and control.

But the teacher is well aware of the difficulties which pupils make for themselves in this procedure, because the immediate call of instinctive habit is so insistent. Pupils must learn to resist that call and develop the power to inhibit, or else they will fall back into their old, harmful habit of blindly pursuing their "end." This means that they forget to give the new directions (the "means"), and fall back again and again for guidance on their unreliable sensory appreciation (feeling).

There are very few adults who are aware of the necessity of *preventing* themselves from falling back into their old subconscious habits, even though the necessity for this is proved to them over and over again. Very few, moreover, have any idea of giving themselves directions without attempting to carry them out. They cannot separate the directions from the acts of which they are the forerunners. Therefore, as soon as they are asked to give the directions to themselves, they rush impulsively into action according to their habitual subconscious use of the parts concerned.

Take, for example, the case of a person who has been accustomed to stiffen his neck muscles in all his daily activities. The teacher points out to him that this habit has come about because he is attempting to make his neck perform the functions of other parts of his mechanism, so that it is not an isolated habit, but is connected with other harmful imperfections in his use of himself. His stiffened neck, in fact, is merely a symptom of general malcoordination: any direct attempt to relax it means that he is dealing with it as if it were a "cause" and not a "symptom." This would result in comparative failure unless a satisfactory co-ordinated use of the mechanism in general is restored. The teacher explains further that, as the pupil's sensory appreciation is unreliable, he is unlikely to be able to remedy these defects by himself, but that if he will inhibit his desire to stiffen his neck, and give himself the new directions to free it, the teacher will be able, by manipulation, to bring about such a general readjustment of his body, that his neck will indeed be freed.

(Note: It is the pupil whose sensory appreciation is most unreliable who is most likely to insist that he really knows what he is doing with himself and will persist in "doing" the mental directions by himself instead of inhibiting this "doing" and allowing the teacher to assist him in the movement which corresponds to the directions.)

If, after this explanation, the pupil directs his neck to be free, the teacher, provided he has the necessary knowledge and experience, will be able to assist him to bring about *those general conditions on which freeing the neck depends.* If, on the other hand, the pupil forgets to inhibit and tries to free his neck directly, he will either do what he has always done with his neck, that is, stiffen it, or he will cause a collapsed condition in some other part or parts, or perhaps in the whole organism. Only when the pupil stops trying to free his neck by direct means will the teacher be able to bring about conditions which make for a satisfactory state of freedom in his neck.

Another difficulty which pupils make for themselves is in connection with the giving of directions. They speak sometimes as if it were a strange and new thing to give themselves directions—forgetting that they have been doing this subconsciously from their earliest days, otherwise they would not be able to stand up without help, much less move about. The point that is new, is that they are asked to direct *consciously* based on a conscious, reasoning use of the organism, the satisfactory employment of which depends on the pupil's clear understanding: (1) as to which of these directions are primary, to be given mentally, but not carried out (inhibition), and (2) as to which are to follow, and to be actually carried out.

To clarify this, let us suppose that the teacher asks the pupil to sit down. If he does so immediately, he will be guided by his unreliable sensory appreciation and will simply repeat his usual faulty subconscious manner of sitting. However, in re-education, as soon as he is asked to sit down he must immediately say "No" and *tell himself not to sit down.* In this way, he will inhibit his usual faulty use of himself associated in the past with this act, and this procedure prevents indulgence in the old subconscious habits.

The pupil then proceeds to give attention to the different guiding directions which the teacher considers essential to the correct control of those psycho-mechanics (the means) concerned with the satisfactory use of the organism as a whole in the act of sitting down.

These are the directions to be ultimately carried out by the pupil.

It follows, then, that the primary directions are to be given and not carried out, and this will prevent the habitual misuse of the mechanism. All directions which follow these preventive ones are to be carried out (at first by the teacher) as they are concerned with the correct "means" of using the mechanism.

I have already pointed out that children, from the first moment of school life onwards, manifest a lack of inhibitory development, and the fact that in most cases they learn to obey orders at once, without stopping to consider the "why and wherefore," is a contributing factor to this harmful condition.

(Note: I know I will be told that if children are to be taught to inhibit, that is, to prevent the misdirected activities, so much time will be taken up with this that they will be unable to get through their studies. Children have said to me, "I could not stop like this in school, they tell us to hurry." I can only say that time spent in teaching children to inhibit impulses to unreasoning activity, to which otherwise they later become slaves, is time not lost, but time actually saved.)

As a result of this early training, many people have become so used to reacting quickly and subconsciously to any stimulus that comes to them that this has become a deep habit which they find difficult to break. In other words, people find it difficult not to want to be obedient, not to want to be right, not to work directly for their end. The difficulty, however, lies not in the thing itself but in the "breaking of a habit" which, if persisted in, makes it impossible for them to achieve a desired end.

It will be found that in every case, a pupil's success in achieving an end, depends on his or her practical recognition of the fact that only by continually attending to the "means" essential to the successful achievement of the "end" can a satisfactory result be secured. This applies equally

(1) whether the pupil is in the early stages of his work, where he is giving directions and leaving the carrying out of these directions to the teacher;

(2) whether she is at a later stage where, under supervision, she is gradually developing a reliable sensory appreciation on which she can rely in carrying out the directions herself, or

(3) whether he is working by himself at his ordinary everyday activities outside.

The above discussion of inhibition leads us to consider the individual's ability to wait (inhibit) before reacting to a stimulus to pursue some "end" in the ordinary way. It may be of interest to give some facts with regard to the experiences of people taking lessons in speaking, breathing, singing, etc.

Most people who need lessons have a tendency to speak too quickly, and they do not pause between their sentences. This tendency has to be checked, but in conscious re-education no attempt is made to check it directly. Therefore, instead of telling the pupil directly to pause, the teacher points out that she is gasping at the end of her sentences, and sniffing or "sucking in air" through the mouth—the result of her incorrect, subconscious conceptions concerned with breathing, and with the incorrect use of the psycho-physical mechanisms as a whole. The pupil must realize that a correct conception of the nature of respiration is essential, together with an understanding of the principles underlying the correct use of the psycho-mechanics involved in the act of breathing, before she makes any attempt to put it into practice.

Only when this point has been reached will the teacher ask the pupil to stop and wait at the end of each sentence, refuse to take another breath until she has inhibited her usual incorrect method of breathing, and substitute for this the new, correct conscious directions which make for increasingly satisfactory use. The teacher therefore asks her to perform:

(1) *an inhibitory act,* that is, to inhibit "my way" of breathing which constitutes the bad habit she has developed when taking breath at the end of each sentence;

(2) *a volitionary act,* that is, to give directions for the means by which a more satisfactory way of breathing may be gradually cultivated, *before she attempts to go on to the next sentence.*

The pupil will very likely object that this pause between sentences will attract attention to herself, because her speech will appear slow and stilted. This objection only means, however, that she does not realize that her old habits of sucking in air through her mouth instead of her nostrils, and running one sentence into another, are noticeable defects to other people. With guidance, these defects will gradually disappear, and the time taken to pause and direct between sentences will become continuously operative, and easier, remaining under the pupil's conscious control. It is unlikely that such defects as these can be eradicated, or the cultivation of new defects prevented, by "breathing exercises" or lessons in "deep-breathing", but if the pupil tackles his difficulties through conscious, constructive re-education he can learn to overcome them.

The above applies equally to singing. The pupil will probably also object that she cannot pause at certain places in a song as she has to keep time. However, this is not so, because when the necessary inhibitory control has been acquired, the pause will only be momentary.

But even if we suppose that the objection holds, what good can it do to keep time if the principles which are essential to good singing—these being the correct and adequate use of the psycho-physical mechanisms connected with respiration—are treated in practice as secondary factors, and are being actually perverted in use?

In all these considerations we must remember that, in attempting to acquire satisfactory psycho-physical functioning, correct use can hardly be at the same speed as that achieved at the cost of an incorrect use of the mechanism. Speed in good use will build up as the necessary experience is gained in lessons.

Now that I have indicated the principles which underlie the general scheme which I advocate for developing a reliable sensory appreciation, I will go on to describe in detail one of the tech nical evolutions (a description of this evolution was first published in 1910) which I use in my teaching. It illustrates what the attitude of the pupil should be towards the practical work involved in developing new sensory appreciation during the performance of the evolution *but, more particularly, as an illustration of the means by which we may develop a reliable sense appreciation of the minimum of so-called "physical tension."* For, in the majority of cases, the most difficult problem to be solved, is that of developing a correct register of the *due and proper amount of so-called "muscular tension" necessary at a given time.*

It is not possible, of course, to tell the pupil the minimum degree of muscle tension required by him or her at any particular moment. And even if this were possible, how could the pupil register this minimum accurately when the very sensory appreciation being used for guidance is unreliable, inaccurate, and often positively delusive?

Probably the most difficult problem from the teacher's point of view, therefore, is this matter of the degree of "physical tension." It clearly cannot be solved simply by performing "physical exercises." Indeed, the main danger of "physical culture exercises" lies in the fact that this fundamental difficulty of muscular tension is ignored. I claim, however, that the problem can be solved in the technical evolution I am about to describe. Please pay special attention to the instructions given to the pupil concerning the use of his or her hands and arms associated with co-ordination, and particularly to the positions of fingers, wrists, and elbows when placed on a chair as directed.

I want it to be very clearly understood that when I write about the arms, legs, hands, feet, etc., *I always imply their co-ordinated use with the body as a co-ordinated support.* Indeed, we might say the body represents the trunk of a tree and the arms the branches.

It must also be clearly understood that in what follows it is taken for granted that the pupil gives special attention to the primary principles laid down by the teacher, before the pupil attempts to carry out any instructions given. If this is done, the majority of the experiences that the pupil receives should be correct ones, thus making for the development of confidence and for the continuance of the processes involved in the eradication of defects.

It is not possible, of course, to give here all the detailed instructions that would meet every case, because these will vary
according to the particular pupil. An experienced teacher, however,
should be able to give these instructions in accordance with the
needs of the individual. We must learn to differentiate between the
variations of the teacher's art and the principles of the teaching
technique being used.

Chapter 4

ILLUSTRATION

In the technical evolution which follows, I am obliged to use certain phrases which must be commented on, because they do not
always adequately express my meaning, and therefore cannot be
defended as being demonstrably accurate.

My reader may ask, then, why I use them. In *Man's Supreme
Inheritance*, I used the phrase "position of mechanical advantage,"
and pointed out that I did so because a better one was not available.
I had sought advice from scientific and literary friends in this connection, and have done so with regard to the phrases which follow.
They are inadequate, but with a teacher present to demonstrate
their meaning, they serve their purpose. The phrases are:

1) SHORTENING OF THE SPINE

One of the most common defects in human beings today is an
undue curving of the spine in the use of the self in the acts of
everyday life, and naturally this causes a shortening in stature. As
a practical demonstration, take a piece of paper, note its length,

then curve it slightly and you will see that its overall length on the vertical is shorter.

2) LENGTHENING OF THE SPINE

If we modify the curve in the spine, we tend to lengthen it, just as the piece of paper will regain its length if stretched out again.

3) RELAX THE NECK

There is considerable confusion on the part of pupils when they attempt to relax some part of the body. In ordinary teaching, pupils and teachers are quite convinced that if some part of the organism is too tense, they can relax it—that is, *do the relaxing by direct means.* This is a delusion, but it is difficult to convince them of it. In the first place, if they do chance to get rid of the specific tension, it will be by a partial collapse of the parts concerned, or possibly even by a general collapse of the whole organism. In the second place, it is obvious that if some part of the organism is unduly tensed, it is because the pupil is attempting to do with it the work of some other part, for which it is quite unsuited.

4) HEAD FORWARD AND UP

This is one of the most inadequate and confusing phrases used as a means of conveying our ideas in words, and it is a dangerous instruction to give to any pupil, unless the teacher first demonstrates to the pupil *by means of manipulation,* the exact experiences involved.

5) WIDEN THE BACK

This instruction rivals the last one in its shortcomings, when considered as a phrase for conveying an idea of what we expect a pupil to construe correctly, unless the teacher is capable of demonstrating what he means by re-adjusting the pupil's organism so that the desired conditions may be brought about.

What really occurs is a very marked change in the position of the bony structures of the thorax, and a permanent enlargement of the thoracic cavity, with a striking increase in thoracic mobility and the minimum muscular tension of the whole of the mechanisms involved.

6) SUPPORT THE BODY WITH THE ARMS

This instruction is given when the pupil is holding the back of a chair, either in sitting or standing, in order to give the teacher the opportunity to pass on quickly and easily certain experiences to the pupil, essential at a particular stage of the work in co-ordination. The varying details of the "means" by which the use indicated by the arms and body is to be gained could not be written down to meet the requirements of each pupil, because they vary with each slight stage of progress. This is why "correct positions" or "postures" have no place in conscious re-education. A "correct position" or "posture" indicates a fixed position, and prevents growth. The correct position today will not be the correct position of next week.

7) WIDEN THE ARMS WHILE SUPPORTING AND RAISING THE BODY

This is the most deceptive of the instructions given in these pages. If it is carried out without manipulative assistance, it is a contradictory instruction, because if the arms are widened, as the act is generally understood, the body would be lowered, not raised. The tendency of the pupil in this movement is to contract unduly the inner muscles of the upper arms, and a skillful teacher can help the pupil to prevent this.

We will now pass on to the illustration.

THE PUPIL IS ASKED TO SIT IN A CHAIR IN ACCORDANCE WITH THE PRINCIPLES SET DOWN IN *Man's Supreme Inheritance*. When he is seated, his body supported by the back of the chair, another chair is placed in front of him with its back towards him.

THE PUPIL IS THEN ASKED TO GIVE THE FOLLOWING PREVENTIVE DIRECTIONS: NOT TO STIFFEN THE NECK, TO DIRECT THE HEAD FORWARD AND UP, TO LENGTHEN THE SPINE.

It must here be clearly understood that in previous manipulative and other work done in the technique, the pupil will have been made familiar with the theory and practice of the first direction, that is, not to stiffen the neck. The pupil is able to give certain

directions correctly and also to carry them out. In the present instance, it is explained to the pupil that the direction given is to be
entirely *preventive*—a projected wish *without any attempt to
carry it out successfully.*

THE TEACHER REPEATS THE DIRECTIONS AND WITH HIS
HANDS HE PROCEEDS TO BRING THE PUPIL'S BODY GENTLY
FORWARD FROM THE HIPS.

It is important to note here that the imperfectly co-ordinated
person tends to *shorten* the stature and *pull the head back* in
making this movement forward. Unless, therefore, the pupil re-
members this subconscious tendency to shorten, and attends to
the counteracting new directions, this old habit will prove too
strong; at the first touch from the teacher, no matter how light or
gentle, the pupil will start to move forward, with, say, perhaps 75%
of subconscious habit and 25% of new conscious response. Even
this estimate is, in most cases, a generous one. Invariably, the pupil
tries to gain the "end" of moving forward, so that the new directions are no longer projected. Instead, the old subconscious habits
still dominate and the pupil stiffens the neck, throws the head back
and shortens the spine by curving it. These particular faults are
accompanied by varying degrees of incorrect tension of the legs
and other parts of the organism, and by a stiffening of the hip
joints. This misuse causes an expenditure of energy out of all proportion to the requirements of the evolution.

When this happens, the teacher must point out that the pupil
has not understood what is required. The teacher must restate the
whole position from as many angles as possible, until the pupil
definitely understands that the primary directions are *preventive.*
The teacher must point out that if the pupil gives these preventive
directions (inhibition) and then proceeds to give the new ones for
moving, *the spine will be kept at its greatest possible length* while
the body is moved forward easily from the hips without interfering
with the generally relative position of the torso, (except in the
matter of the angle), just as a door moves on its hinges.

THE TEACHER WILL THEN RENEW THE REQUEST TO THE

PUPIL TO GIVE HIS DIRECTIONS AND WITH HIS HANDS WILL DO THE ACTUAL MOVEMENT FOR THE PUPIL. Sometimes the pupil can request the teacher to move his (the pupil's) body forward while he (the pupil) gives his directions. When the teacher is satisfied that the pupil is giving adequate attention to the directions up to this point, and appreciates their relative value as primary, secondary, and following factors; and when the correct sensory experiences, made possible by the teacher's guidance, have been sufficiently repeated, the pupil can then be taken a step further.

At every step, it is essential that the pupil rehearses the directions from the beginning, because these earlier directions constitute the *means* by which a further step may be successfully taken. In giving themselves directions, pupils must on every occasion begin with the primary ones before going on to the secondary, and so on.

THE PUPIL MUST NOW AGAIN DIRECT THE NECK NOT TO STIFFEN AND THE HEAD FORWARD AND UP, WHILE THE TEACHER SECURES WITH HIS HANDS THAT POSITION OF THE TORSO IN WHICH THE BACK IS WIDENED.

These directions should be repeated several times and be *continued* WHILE THE TEACHER TAKES THE PUPIL'S RIGHT ARM AND MOVES IT FORWARD UNTIL THE PUPIL'S HAND IS ABOVE THE TOP RAIL OF THE BACK OF THE CHAIR. THE PUPIL SHOULD THEN BE ASKED TO REPEAT THE DIRECTIONS, AND THEN TO TAKE THE WEIGHT OF THE ARM ENTIRELY AS THE TEACHER DISENGAGES HIS HANDS FROM THE SUPPORTED ARM.

Great care must be taken to see that the pupil has not interfered with the mechanism of the torso in the effort to take the weight of the arm. Interference implies that the pupil has forgotten his or her directions and has fallen back into subconscious habits. What is essential here, is a *co-ordinated use* of the arms. The only way to achieve this is by first giving the necessary preventive directions, and then rehearsing the new directions given by the teacher, in which the movement of the arms is linked up with the use of other parts of the body.

If the pupil has not interfered with the torso in taking the weight of the arm, HE SHOULD NEXT BE ASKED TO GRASP THE TOP RAIL OF THE BACK OF THE CHAIR GENTLY AND FIRMLY, KEEPING THE FINGERS AS STRAIGHT AS POSSIBLE, FLAT AGAINST THE FRONT OF THE TOP RAIL. THE THUMB SHOULD ALSO BE AS STRAIGHT AS POSSIBLE AGAINST THE BACK OF THE TOP RAIL, WITH THE WRIST CURVED SLIGHTLY INWARDS.

If, however, the pupil fails to continue to give his or her directions, *the pupil must be requested to begin once more at the very first step, and the whole process repeated until a satisfactory result has been secured.* It should be realized that in doing this repeatedly a process of fundamental sensory building is going on, on a general and not a specific basis.

THE PUPIL MUST THEN BE ASKED AGAIN TO DIRECT THE NECK NOT TO STIFFEN, THE HEAD TO GO FORWARD AND UP; AND THE TEACHER WILL REPEAT HIS PREVIOUS EFFORT TO ESTABLISH THAT CONDITION OF THE TORSO AND BACK ESSENTIAL TO SATISFACTORY ARM WORK. THE PROCEDURE IS THEN REPEATED WITH THE LEFT ARM, SO THAT THE PUPIL WILL BE GRASPING THE BACK OF THE CHAIR WITH BOTH HANDS.

Some pupils will, of course, need more assistance in this than others. The decision as to when and how much help is needed must be left to the discretion of the teacher. *To achieve success, correct experiences in sensory appreciation must follow the giving of directions. By the repetition of this process, the pupils reach a stage where they can depend on themselves with confidence.*

AT THIS POINT THE PUPIL SHOULD BE ASKED TO RECONSIDER THE DIFFERENT *MEANS* BY WHICH HE HAS REACHED THIS STAGE, AND TO REPEAT ORALLY THE DIRECTIONS EXACTLY IN THE SEQUENCE GIVEN TO HIM BY THE TEACHER AS PRIMARY, SECONDARY, AND FOLLOWING FACTORS. In this way the teacher will be able to test the pupil's accuracy or otherwise in this connection. *While the pupil repeats the directions, he must remain in the co-ordinated condition which has been secured during the performance of the evolution.*

When the teacher is satisfied that the pupil has succeeded up to this point, he or she may give the pupil additional guiding directions which are:

(1) TO CONTINUE TO HOLD THE TOP RAIL OF THE CHAIR WITH STRAIGHT FINGERS AS PREVIOUSLY DESCRIBED;
(2) TO ALLOW THE WRISTS TO BE CURVED INWARDS;
(3) TO ALLOW THE ELBOWS TO BE CURVED OUTWARDS.

In order to keep holding the rail in this way, THE PUPIL SHOULD REHEARSE GIVING ALL THE DIRECTIONS PREVIOUSLY TOLD HIM AND WHICH HE HAS ALREADY ORALLY REPEATED TO THE TEACHER.

The teacher's aim is now to give the pupil the experiences necessary to a gentle, forearm pull from the fingers, and to this end WILL TAKE HOLD OF THE PUPIL'S ELBOWS AND DIRECT THEM OUTWARDS AND SLIGHTLY DOWNWARDS, and then, following this, will give the sensory experiences required in DIRECTING THE UPPER PARTS OF THE ARMS (ABOVE THE ELBOW) AWAY FROM ONE ANOTHER IN SUCH A WAY THAT THE PUPIL WILL BE SUPPORTING THE TORSO WITH HIS ARMS.

THE PUPIL IS NOW ASKED TO CONTINUE TO SUPPORT THE TORSO IN THIS WAY, CONTINUING ALSO TO REHEARSE HIS DIRECTIONS, while the teacher adjusts the torso in such a way that the large "lifting" muscles of the back will be employed co-ordinately with the other parts of the organism to bring about such use of the respiratory mechanisms that they will function to the maximum at the particular stage of development reached from day to day. Success in this part of the evolution will bring about a change in the condition of the back which would be described by the ordinary observer as a "widening of the back."

These directions are the *means* by which such use of the mechanisms may be brought about, associated with a satisfactory re-adjustment of the back, as will cause the floating ribs to move freely, and also tend to develop the maximum intra-thoracic capacity and to establish the most effective use of the respiratory mechanism during the sleeping as well as the waking hours.

Let me take the opportunity here to set down some of the impeding conditions which are present in most pupils during this evolution. For instance, the muscular tension employed in using the fingers and arms is usually a harmful and unnecessary one. Often, the undue tension of the arm muscles prevents the pupil from using the fingers to the best advantage in holding the chair. I have known instances where the fingers are actually held away from the wood without the pupil knowing it. This undue tension is particularly noticeable in the contractor muscles in the region of the biceps and in the pectoral muscles in the front of the chest. In a satisfactory state of sensory appreciation these muscles would remain more or less relaxed and the greater part of the work would fall on the muscles of the opposite side of the arms and the back (chiefly the latissimus dorsi). This situation makes for both the maximum activity of the respiratory mechanisms, with the minimum effort, and also for an increased intra-thoracic capacity, accompanied by a broadening of the costal arch (increased vital capacity).

Other impeding conditions are likely to occur at the pupil's first attempts to pull with the arms. In his attempt to do this, either one or other or all of the fingers will become bent and the wrists will be curved outwards, *exactly the reverse of the action indicated by the directions and of the one desired. This failure to carry out the given directions is due chiefly to the fact that the pupil's sensory appreciation in the matter of the necessary muscular tension is sadly inadequate.*

This leads us directly to a consideration of the means we have adopted in order to develop the pupil's reliable sensory appreciation, the *means* by which he or she will perform this evolution with the *minimum of muscular tension.* The reader's attention is specially directed to the following:

If the pupil will carry out the act of the forearm pull and attend to the widening of the upper parts of the arms, while continuing to recognize the keeping of the fingers straight and the wrists curved inwards as primary factors, *the minimum tension will be exerted.* As soon as the pupil interferes with the position of the fingers or wrists (curving wrists outwards instead of inwards), this will indicate that *the point of minimum muscular tension has been passed.*

It should be noted here that the pupil's position in this act is an ideal one for watching the hands and wrists. Therefore, if the pupil will watch carefully any tendency to make incorrect movements, these can be prevented at once. However, it will again be seen that many pupils are unable to "keep watch," and depend instead on the old haphazard method of "trying to do it right," guided by feeling—feeling which, in the past, has proved unreliable.

There has just come to my knowledge an interesting objection to the importance which I attach to the process of inhibition as a primary and fundamental factor in conscious control. The objection is that inhibition will cause harmful suppression in the individual concerned. I will, therefore, show that this objection is based on a complete misunderstanding of the fundamental principles and processes involved in my technique.

There is a growing tendency to attempt to free children from undue external restraint, both at home and at school, in order to prevent those harmful suppressions and inhibitions which are now considered to have been caused by the imposition of the restraint prevalent in past methods. The points I wish to make are: (1) that the kind of inhibition involved here is directly linked with the idea of gaining a specific end, that is, of controlling a child's response to a stimulus arising from some primary desire or need, and, (2) and this is most important, that the stimulus to inhibit this response comes from without, and is therefore *forced* on the pupil through a command from an outside authority. This could account for the disturbed emotional conditions associated with what is known as suppression.

The inhibitory process involved in my technique has little in common with the process mentioned above. In my technique, inhibition is conceived on a general and preventive basis and is employed primarily in connection with ideas which are dissociated from any direct attempt to gain an "end." Instead it involves that indirect procedure inseparable from the practical application of the principle of the "means" by which an "end" may be gained. These ideas are the response to a stimulus arising from reasoned, constructive, conscious understanding by the pupil of the principles concerning the "means"; the application of these principles prevents "end-gaining" acts, which are usually associated with misdirected activities. If the pupil accepts the need and efficacy of working with the "means" used to do something, it follows that he or she must accept the principle of inhibition of primary desires in "end-gaining" acts. (Primary desires are simply the "ends" we wish to achieve). This means that in my technique, inhibition—that is, *the act of refusing to respond* to the primary desire to gain an "end"—*becomes the act of responding (volitionary act)* to the conscious reasoned desire to employ the *means* of gaining that "end."

The stimulus to inhibit, therefore, in this case, comes from within and is not forced on the pupil. This means that the pupil's desires will be satisfied, not thwarted, and that desirable emotional and other psycho-physical conditions will be present which do not make for what is known as suppression in any form.

(Note: Many people pride themselves on self-control, but they are really victims of enslavement to a fixed "end." They do not control themselves by stopping to think out the "means" to their "ends," but by excluding everything which does not agree with the "ends" which they have set up as right and proper. They may contend that their control is self-imposed and not externally imposed, but to other people it appears to be a form of rigidity—a rigidity which is inseparable from enslavement to preconceived and unreasoned ideas of what is right and proper in conduct and procedure.)

The tendency of people to speak and act on a subconscious plane without adequate thought or consideration is a particularly marked manifestation when an unusually powerful stimulus is present to those processes known as prejudice and emotional disturbances. We are all familiar with the phrases, "Why don't you think before you act?" "Think before you speak," and so on. When the human being's activities are on a plane of constructive, conscious control, that individual will be able to apply the principle of inhibition in his or her activities in the outside world just as they have applied it to their psycho-physical self, with accruing benefit in both spheres of application.

Here is an example of the application of the technique to the practical ways of life. It shows the analogy that exists between "linking-up" (association of ideas) during the lessons, and linking-up what has been gained in those lessons with the experience of everyday life.

A pupil of mine, an author, had been in a serious state of health for some time, and could no longer carry on with his literary work. He had what was described as a "breakdown," and as a result, even a few hours work caused him great fatigue and depression. From the beginning of his lessons, therefore, I stipulated that he should work for half an hour at most, and then *stop* and either do fifteen minutes work in respiratory re-education, or take a walk in the open air before resuming work.

One day he arrived for his lesson unusually depressed and admitted that he had been working non-stop for four hours. I pointed out that it was hardly surprising that he was in such a state, because when one is in deep thought, the breathing is reduced to a minimum, just as in sleep. This minimum was particularly harmful in his case because of the inadequacy of his intra-thoracic capacity which was one of the symptoms that caused his "breakdown." "But I can't stop once I am into my work," he objected. I told him that if this were so, it must be due to some lack of control on his part. "But surely, it is a mistake to break my train of thought?" he objected further. I answered that on the contrary, it should be just as easy to break off from work requiring thought, as it is to carry on a train of thought while taking a walk with all its attendant interruptions. It should also be possible to find the connection again easily on returning to the work but with the accompanying benefit to the individual.

In this, I was preparing the way to showing this pupil the analogy that existed between the point in question and his difficulty in accomplishing certain simple parts of the technique in his lessons, through his disinclination to stop. I wished to convince him that *the gaining of control in the simple psycho-physical evolutions done during lessons means sooner or later the gaining of control in everyday activities.*

In this, however, he was only like thousands of other well-educated, intelligent people who, in dealing with a situation, fail to make an obvious association of ideas, and so miss important connecting links. In this case, had he made the necessary connection between the difficulty he had in "stopping" in his lessons, and "stopping" in his outside activities, this recognition would have given a new meaning and an added stimulus to the psycho-physical effort on which the successful working-out of the technique depends.

Chapter 5

RESPIRATORY MECHANISMS

We will probably find the best practical illustration of the need for correct sensory experiences in guidance and control if we consider sensory appreciation in its connection with the psycho-mechanics of respiration. It is universally admitted that harmful defects exist in the way most people breathe. Scientific medicine describes certain types of children as born with a "low respiratory need"; this really means that when the child is born it is imperfectly co-ordinated and its organism is functioning much nearer to the minimum than to the maximum capacity. This condition prevails in most people today, and is commonly known as "bad-breathing." However, so-called "bad-breathing" is only a symptom and not a primary cause of the malcondition, because the standard of breathing depends on the standard of general co-ordinated use of the psycho-physical mechanisms. People are not "bad-breathers," they are poorly co-ordinated.

A "bad-breather" is usually recommended to adopt "breathing exercises" or take "lessons in breathing" in order to "cure" the symptom; but this, once more, is an example of specifically trying to gain an "end." As in so many other spheres, a vicious circle is developed.

Let me attempt to make this clear. Open any book on breathing, either by a scientist or an expert in vocal or "physical culture," and read the instructions for the exercises recommended in it. Or look at children or adults in a gymnasium being taught breathing and you will see proof of attempts at improvement on a specific rather than a general basis, all alike based on the same "end-gaining" principles.

People are taught to take deep breaths and perhaps to perform some "physical" movement at the same time in an attempt to increase the chest expansion. Yet it is a scientific fact that all "physical" tension tends to cause thoracic rigidity and breathlessness, two conditions which should be avoided by people who are attempting to pass from "bad breathing" to satisfactory respiratory functioning.

Specific defects to be noted when watching pupils during their attempts at "deep-breathing" have already been set down in *Man's Supreme Inheritance*. Here we will deal only with the defective *general* use of the psycho-physical organism during these attempts. In order to make the point, we must refer to the fact that the pupil and the teacher must have recognized certain harmful manifestations which called for some remedial procedure on the lines of "deep-breathing," etc. These harmful manifestations would be the result of misuse of the organism.

Certain incorrect uses of the mechanism have become established, associated with unreliable sensory appreciation; and any effort to correct this by "deep-breathing" or any other "lessons in breathing" is merely an attempt to cure a *general* defective condition of psycho-mechanics by a *specific* remedy. In other words, the same unreliable sensory awareness present at the start of the attempt, is used for guidance in doing the exercises. If practice in breathing exercises continues, therefore, the original defects in the general use of the mechanism will become more pronounced and will even increase in number.

It may be argued that the pupil's chest size is increased as a result of these lessons, that he "feels better," etc. This may be so, but due to the unreliability of his sensory awareness, what he feels is likely to be a delusion. Of what good is "feeling better" if one is still left guided by defective sensory appreciation? In time he will discover that other serious conditions have developed. We have all known people who tell of improvement in their chest measurements as a result of exercises, but this is mainly due to muscular development on the outside of the chest rather than co-ordinated expansion of the thoracic capacity. It is the same when people say they "feel better" as a result of breathing exercises: the expert observer can see that the habit of sniffing in air, contraction of the alae nasi, depression of the larynx, and all the accompanying defective use of the organism in doing the exercises must eventually cause serious nose, ear, eye, and throat troubles. In other words, the exponents of breathing exercises act in direct pursuance of their "end" and remain oblivious to the harm caused by the "means" which they use to achieve this "end," and to the many wrong uses cultivated during the process.

If we consider the problem from the point of view of conscious re-education and the fundamental principles underlying the act of breathing, we will see that breathing is very far removed from the primary principle concerned, and that it is, therefore, incorrect and harmful to speak of "teaching a person to breathe," or "giving lessons in breathing." Such a stimulus at once induces projections of all the established incorrect concepts associated with inadequate breathing; it sets all our bad breathing habits in motion.

Breathing is that psycho-physical act by which air is taken into and expelled from the lungs. The lungs consist of two bags containing a network of cells capable of contraction and expansion, with air passages and blood vessels so arranged that oxygen can be absorbed through the tissue of the blood vessels, cells, and air passages whilst carbonic acid gas (poison) passes through this tissue from the blood vessels into lung cells to be expelled from the lungs. The bony thorax consists of the spinal vertebrae, the ribs, and the sternum. The ribs attached to the sternum and the spine are much less mobile than the lower "floating" ribs, which are not attached to the sternum. The lungs are enclosed in the thorax of which the diaphragm is the floor, and the only entrance to which is through the trachea (wind-pipe). From the very first breath, there is a more or less constant air pressure (atmospheric pressure) within the lungs, but no pressure on the outside of the lungs. Air pressure is sufficient to overcome the elasticity of the tissue of the air-cells, and to increase their size when not held in check by the pressure of the thorax on the lung-bag itself. The lungs are subject, however, to this pressure from the thoracic walls during contraction, and to the release of this pressure during expansion of the thoracic cavity. The pressure that can be exerted by the thoracic walls on the outside of the lung-bag is much greater than that which is exerted by the atmospheric pressure within the lungs. Therefore, when we wish, as we say, to "take a breath" (inspiration), we reduce the pressure exerted on the lungs by the thoracic walls, and employ those muscular co-ordinations which increase the intra-thoracic capacity of the lungs. This causes a partial vacuum in the lung cells of which atmospheric pressure takes advantage, by increasing the size of the cells and thus the amount of air in the lungs. If, then, we wish to exhale (expiration), we merely have to increase the pressure on the lungs by contracting the thoracic walls, which overcomes atmospheric pressure in the lungs and forces the air out. During these contractions and expansions the diaphragm moves up and down in harmony with the adjustments of the thoracic walls.

The foregoing should convince the reader that if anyone wishes to secure the maximum control and development in breathing, one has to be able to command the maximum functioning of the psycho-physical mechanisms concerned with the satisfactory expansion and contraction of the thoracic walls. *It is not necessary even to think of taking a breath;* in fact, it is harmful to do so when the mechanism is in a condition requiring re-education.

The crux of the matter, then, is to gain this control in expanding and contracting the chest, and thus permanently to increase its capacity and mobility. This calls for a comprehensive consideration of the primary, secondary, and other psycho-physical factors involved.

Naturally, the most powerful stimulus to the use of the respiratory mechanisms is the need for oxygen and the elimination of carbonic acid gas from the blood. But we must remember that the pupil's incorrect use of the mechanism is an impeding factor in achieving the desired control and the increased thoracic capacity. Therefore, the first objective is to *prevent the psycho-physical activities which are responsible for this defective use,* through the pupil's ability to inhibit. The teacher must correctly diagnose the pupil's numerous bad habits of breathing in everyday life, and have a comprehensive understanding of the faulty sensory appreciation, conception, adjustment, and co-operation which are manifested in these bad habits.

The teacher should explain this to the pupil, and then give him or her a reasoned consideration of the "means" of improving co-ordination. The pupil is taught to inhibit, by giving the preventive guiding directions, the deceptive guiding sensations involved with the bad habits in breathing. The teacher must make certain that the directions *are given by the pupil in the sequence in which they are to be employed.* The pupil may then begin the practice of prevention. He or she must repeatedly refuse to try for an "end," positively pause to think of the original faults pointed out by the teacher, and refuse to repeat them.

For instance, suppose that a male pupil has a special desire to increase his chest capacity. This desire acts as a stimulus to the psycho-physical processes involved and sets off all the unreliable sensations associated with his established idea of chest expansion. He must *refuse to act* on this idea. He must *definitely stop* and say to himself: "No, I won't do what I should like to do to increase my chest capacity because, if I do what I feel will increase it, I will only use my mechanisms as I have used them before, and what good is that?" In other words, he inhibits his desire to act.

The teacher, of course, must decide when the pupil should proceed from the purely preventive to the next stage of work. The teacher then names the new directions needed for the satisfactory guiding sensations concerned with the correct use of the mechanisms involved. The pupil should give himself these new directions while the teacher, by manipulation, helps him to secure satisfactory experiences which should be repeated until the bad habits are eradicated.

Repetition of these correct experiences establishes a satisfactory use of the mechanism so that an increase or decrease of the chest capacity can be secured at will and with the minimum of effort. The increase in intra-thoracic capacity decreases the pressure on the outside of the lung-bag, causing a momentary partial vacuum in the lungs, which is promptly filled with air because of the atmospheric pressure exerted on the inside of the lung-cells. This increases the amount of air in the lungs and constitutes the act of "taking a breath" (inspiration). The marvelous efficiency of the respiratory machine, when properly used, becomes apparent when we realize that we have only to employ the same "means" by which we secure the increase to secure the decrease of the intra-thoracic capacity. In this act, the contracting chest walls exert such increased pressure on the lungs that the air-pressure within is overcome, expelling the air (expiration). Inspiration and expiration make up the complete act of breathing. When satisfactory breathing is achieved, the teacher may then proceed to help the pupil to employ this co-ordinated use in connection with all vocal effort. This should begin with *whispered* vocalization—preferably the vowel sound "Ah," as this form of vocal use is so rarely used in everyday life and is, therefore, rarely associated with ordinary bad psycho-physical habits in speaking, singing, etc.

For this reason, the teacher begins by helping the pupil to make an expiration on a whispered "Ah." This calls for a knowledge of the psycho-physical "means" in using the organism *in general,* and of the acts of opening the mouth, using the lips, tongue, soft palate, etc., with freedom from stress and strain in the vocal mechanisms. To this end a definite technique is employed. This technique prevents sniffing and "sucking in air," undue depression of the larynx, and undue stiffening of the muscles of the throat, vocal organs, and neck. It also prevents the undue lifting of the front of the chest during inspiration, its undue depression during expiration, and also many other defects which are developed by any imperfectly co-ordinated person who attempts to learn "breathing" or "deep breathing," etc., while guided by the unreliable sensory appreciation which is always associated with imperfect use of the psycho-physical mechanism.

Chapter 6

UNDULY EXCITED FEAR REFLEXES, UNCONTROLLED EMOTIONS, AND FIXED PREJUDICES

There can be little doubt that the process of reasoning tends to develop more quickly and to reach a higher standard in a person whose attitude towards life is calm and collected. In such a person, psycho-physical habits are governed by moderation, and the powers of inhibition are adequately developed. These inhibitory powers are not limited to those comparatively few areas of life where it was considered necessary to establish taboos during humankind's struggle with the problems that arose during the development of civilization. In these areas where taboos exist, there has been a harmful and exaggerated development of inhibition, often causing virtues to become vices. In other areas there has been a correspondingly harmful lack of inhibition, particularly in relation to the use of the psycho-physical mechanisms in practical activities. This unbalanced use of this wonderful process of inhibition tends to cause unbalanced functioning throughout the organism and establishes what I refer to as "the unduly excited reflex" process.

This unbalanced state is apparent in civilized humans, and the child of today is more predisposed to this condition than its parents or ancestors. Children, therefore, start their school career with poor inhibitory powers. Now, volition and inhibition are invaluable birthrights of the human creature *and should be developed equally;* but from the first moment of school life right up to adolescence, the child's training tends to interfere with balanced development.

(Note: The fact of the great number of "don'ts" to which some children are subjected, and the implicit obedience expected of them at school, does not affect my contention that the children of today manifest a serious lack of inhibition in their use of themselves.)

Unduly excited fear reflexes, uncontrolled emotions, prejudices, and fixed habits are retarding factors in all human development. They need our serious attention, because they are linked up with all psycho-physical processes employed in growth and development on the subconscious plane. By the time adolescence is reached, these retarding factors have become present in varying degrees, and the processes established in psycho-physical use will make for the continued development of such retarding factors. This is particularly true when a person attempts to learn something calling for new experiences.

If one watches adult pupils at their lessons, it becomes clear that uncontrolled emotions are a striking feature in their attempts to carry out new instructions correctly. They will tend to have fixed expressions and jerky uncontrolled movements; they hold their breath by adopting harmful postures, exerting harmful stress and strain, as though they were performing strenuous "physical" acts. In many cases twitching occurs in the muscles of the mouth and cheeks, or fingers. This is because pupils think they must try to do *correctly* what the teacher asks, and, on the subconscious plane, the teacher does insist on this. The teacher of re-education on a conscious plane, however, does not insist on this—because he or she knows that where there is a faulty functioning of the organism, *individuals cannot always do what they are asked to do correctly.* They may "want" to do it, they may "try and try again"; but as long as the psycho-mechanics they employ are not working satisfactorily they can have only partial success. Their judgment is based on delusive sensory appreciation and they are stuck in the vicious circle of their old habits as long as they try to do things "correctly." Paradoxically, the pupil's only chance of success lies not in "trying to be right," but in "wanting to be wrong" —wrong, that is, by his or her own standard. Every unsuccessful "try" reinforces the old wrong psycho-physical habits associated with the pupil's conception of a particular act; it involves at the same time new emotional experiences of discouragement, fear, and anxiety, so that wrong experiences and unduly excited fear reflexes become one in the pupil's recognition. They "make the food they feed on" —and the more conscientious teacher and pupil are on this plan, the worse the situation becomes for both.

This is why a teacher on a conscious plane does not expect a pupil to perform any new act "correctly," but instead, uses his hands to give repeated new experiences to the pupil until they become established. The pupil is asked to stop "end-gaining" and to attend to the guiding directions which are the "means," the "how," of doing, until one day the "end" may be gained. This will take time; but eventually the pupil will be able to repeat the act with precision at all times and under all circumstances, because unduly excited fear reflexes, uncontrolled emotions, and fixed prejudices will not have been developed in the process just outlined. Indeed, it is a process which does not involve the teacher asking the pupils to perform any act until their sensory appreciation has improved to the point where they can do so with ease. This breeds confidence and eliminates emotional disturbances which tend towards the minimum instead of the maximum functioning.

The relation of all this to the very important question of the ability to "keep one's head" at critical moments is clear. So let us apply the foregoing points to playing games and other performances in which skill and "presence of mind" are required. We constantly hear remarks like "I didn't do so badly at first, but the more I play the worse I play." A reporter says that it is a curious feature of golf that "the more one knows about it . . . the more difficult it seems to become"; and a well-known professional confessed that golf had become almost too much for him. All this applies equally to other games. I have chosen golf for my illustration because writers on golf unwittingly emphasize the existence of a *problem* underlying such admissions. For instance, they have commented on the failure of some top player to perform a simple stroke at a crucial point when success depends on not throwing a chance away. They have also observed that some players hurry their strokes through anxiety to "get it over." "Truly heart-breaking" is the description of one such incident, words that are echoed by many who have had similar experiences in other matters besides golf.

We are told this is all caused by "nerves." It is undoubtedly a case of the undue excitement of fear reflexes on the player's part—fear that she may miss a shot which she knows she is not in the habit of missing. A pupil once said to me, "I always come up against things I know I can do, and yet when it comes to the point, I can't do them." The fact is that, in learning things, our fear reflexes are unduly excited by the teaching methods used—according to which demands are made on us which we cannot meet. So for a time we get bad results, with the undue and harmful development of emotional reflex processes which inevitably accompany these unsuccessful attempts. We continue to practice on wrong lines, so that successes are few and failures many. We attempt sub-consciously to develop a particular stroke, and in the failure to make the stroke successfully the imperfect use of the psycho-physical mechanism plays a large part. These experiences cause disappointment, unduly excited fear reflexes, and serious emo-tional disturbances—and nothing is done at this later stage to nullify the effects of the psycho-physical experiences cultivated during the earlier stages. These emotional disturbances were part and parcel of an unbalanced psycho-physical condition, a state of anxiety and confusion, and there is no doubt that any unusual incident will bring about a recurrence of the same anxieties which occurred in the early stages of learning.

Only a small minority of experts really know *how* they get their results and effects. With the majority, if anything puts them "off their game," they experience considerable difficulty in getting back on to it again.

(Note: The same applies to expert singers who do not know how they sing, any more than the political and social leaders know how much they are influenced in their actions by their fixed prejudices and emotional gusts, rather than by their reasoning processes.)

Only by having a clear conception of what is required to make a successful stroke or other act, and a knowledge of the "means," can there be any certainty of attaining sureness and confidence during performance.

All that I have written here has been endorsed by that dis-tinguished golfer Mr. John Duncan Dunn, and this is a matter of great gratification to me. I pointed out in my earlier volume that the success of any process in golf, such as "following through," depends primarily on the standard of the *general* use of the mechanism—because a player whose sensory appreciation is faulty cannot satisfactorily carry out directions given to him.

Reliable sensory appreciation is the indispensable preliminary to success. Satisfactory *general* use is essential to satisfactory *specific* use: You may make a good stroke by chance without having good use, but you can never be certain of repeating it; and this uncertainty does not make confidence grow, but rather develops undue fear reflexes and emotional disturbances.

(Note: Here is a delightful little parable from *The Times*, October 29th, 1921, which shows the fallacy of expecting people to put right some defect unless the "means" of doing so is given into their hands first of all:

On the golf course, I met two elderly men playing a short hole. No. 1 had a good shot on to the green, No. 2 did not.

"How can such things be?" No. 2 exclaimed.

No. 1 replied complacently, "I could put you right in a minute."

I waited, breathless, thinking that at last the secret of all hitting was about to be revealed.

"You don't follow through," said No. 1.

It was yet one more disappointment in a bitterly disappointed life, *because I knew that I, and most other people, very often "don't follow through," and that this knowledge does not make me play any better.*

"Oh No. 1," I murmured, "what is the good of telling me that? You must tell me what *I do with my confounded arms and legs on the way up, that makes them behave so badly on the way down.* You are not such a good coach after all, No. 1."

I went away sorrowful.)

We must realize that if an individual is to reach that satisfactory stage of progress in using himself, where he can be reasonably certain of successfully achieving his "ends," he must attend to the "means" to be adopted—regardless of whether the performance is correct or incorrect—during progress in the activities concerned. Application of these principles in any field of learning means that during lessons the teacher must be able to supply the pupil's needs in the matter of reliable sensory appreciation, by giving the necessary experiences from day to day until they become established.

Any technique which does not meet the demands indicated here will prove unsatisfactory as a means of re-educating a pupil on a general basis to a reliable plane of conscious activity. When this plane is reached, the individual comes to rely on the "means" and does not become disturbed by wondering whether the activity be right or wrong. Confidence increases with experiences which are not associated with over-excited fear reflexes and is reinforced by achieving reliable sensory appreciation, which ensures that any interference with the co-ordinated use of oneself will come to one's attention as soon as it occurs (awareness). This confidence associated with awareness is not likely to fail you in moments of crisis, but will prove your protector and reliable guide. You will remember at such moments to reason and to judge, and the resultant judgment, being based on experiences gained through reliable sensory appreciation, will be sound.

I would like now to discuss the matter of unduly excited fear reflexes in connection with processes used in tests made on children in school.

In some schools special mechanical tests are made in order to "grade" the children. The child's "mental apparatus" is, as it were, put on the rack and his or her intellectual status and educational fate probably depend on the results. The tests are supposed to be a reliable guide as to the line of procedure to be taken in the child's school education, and to the particular career he or she will later be advised to follow.

A teacher recently told me of an interesting experience in this connection. She visited a school where a psychologist was testing the children for qualities of accuracy, muscular control, observation, etc. A seven-year-old boy who had shown various symptoms described as "nervous" was waiting to be tested for "control." The test was to enable the authorities to prescribe a curriculum to suit his special needs. An electrical apparatus was placed before the boy.

It consisted of a metal tray with rows of holes in it, decreasing gradually in size. He was told to touch the center of each hole with a pencil-like rod. If he made a mistake and touched the side of the hole, an electric flash occurred.

The child, having already started in a state of nervous dread, became so excited *through the fear of making a mistake* that his hand shook and he stiffened his whole body. This caused the rod to touch the side of the first hole, making him still more afraid. As he became more fearful, he failed to do any hole successfully. Such a test, taken with such emotional conditions, is not a reliable guide to anyone wishing to estimate his potentialities. Indeed, I can prove that nine out of ten children are imperfectly co-ordinated and a great number have serious psycho-physical defects.

Compare the animate human organism to the inanimate machine—say, a car. Would any sane person test a car on the road if he knew that a number of important parts were wrongly adjusted? And if he did, could he expect to judge the standard of functioning of that make of car by the test? Certainly not! Unfortunately, this same idea does not prevail in education. The "end-gaining" principle still dominates, and reasoning about co-ordinated psycho-physical functioning plays little part.

The first need of the imperfectly controlled child is to be consciously re-adjusted until the standard of functioning of the organism is satisfactory. The organism will then function as near to the maximum as is possible, and functioning will continue to improve as the child gradually develops to a standard of conscious guidance in its use, which sets up the conditions essential to the development of latent potentialities.

We have all heard of wonderful feats being performed by people in an emotional state; of "faith cures" being effected when the subjects of these "cures" are in that uncontrolled and harmful psycho-physical state similar to drunkenness or mild insanity. I know a man who never accomplished anything until he was half-crazed with alcohol. I also know of a carriage painter who cannot paint straight lines unless he is drunk. There are many instances of people performing remarkable acts while in an uncontrolled emotional state in which they have been a danger to themselves and to those around them. Men are sent into battle half-drunk so that their "controls" may be temporarily released, and for centuries bands of musicians have been employed in warfare to induce this emotional condition of lowered control. "Muddling through by instinct " is unintelligent enough, but deliberately to induce a condition of lowered control through artificial means (such as are used for example in "faith cure," auto-suggestion, religious revivalism, etc.) is an insult to even a very lowly evolved intelligence. The borderland of insanity is reached through such means, and if these psycho-physical experiences involved are repeated sufficiently, madness will follow. In all these instances the "end-gaining" principle prevails, and the people subjected to these unnatural and harmful experiences are influenced by them for the rest of their lives, because these uncontrolled forces are rarely mastered again. They recur to a lesser or greater extent in other activities and frequently develop into dangerous manifestations, culminating often in tragedy. If a person is dominated by uncontrolled emotions, even a weak stimulus will cause him to indulge in dangerous activities. The repetition of such experiences is the beginning of the formation of what we call a habit, in this case the habit of unbalanced psycho-physical activity. Unfortunately, it does not take long to establish a bad habit.

(Note: Worry is one such habit which is very hard to break. Often, curiously, although the cause of the worry is removed, the habit does not stop. The person himself manufactures the stimulus to worry.)

So-called "mental" tricks are more common than "physical" ones, and when indulged in, soon become habitual. Indulgence in one bad habit tends to lead to the development of others, with a rapid increase in the degree of indulgence.

We must recognize the fact that the human creature cannot be expected to control bad habits unless he or she possesses reliable sensory appreciation and satisfactory use of the mechanisms involved. No form of discipline or other outside influence can secure that satisfactory standard of functioning necessary for control either within or without the organism.

One who lacks this control needs to be re-educated on a general basis to restore reliable sensory appreciation and the desired satisfactory use of the mechanism. Re-education demands that the "means" to any "end" must be reasoned out. With continued use of these reasoning processes, uncontrolled impulses and "emotional gusts" will gradually cease to dominate, and will ultimately be dominated. The organism will not then be called on to satisfy those unhealthy cravings associated with unreliable and delusive sensory appreciation (debauched kinesthesia).

Reasoning out the "means" of gaining "ends" simply implies a commonsense approach. Common sense is a very familiar term, and we all have our particular conception of what it means. Indeed, individual opinion in regard to the meaning of "common sense" can differ as much as it does in regard to religion, politics, social, and educational matters. I will, therefore, put my point of view regarding common sense by giving an example where a person does not show common sense. The man who suffers from digestive and liver disorders, and knows that the cause is too much drinking, or excessive eating, and who still continues to indulge despite the suffering he is causing himself, and despite the advice of his doctor to cut down, cannot be said to be acting with common sense.

The reader may say that the man is unable to stop over-indulging. Let us consider this inability. Firstly, it is clear that the man had recognized that he was ill because he had consulted his doctor. This proves that the stimulus had reached his consciousness, and no doubt he was prepared to take medical treatment, provided it did not interfere with his habit of over-indulging. But, of course, he cannot become healthy again using such an unreasoning procedure. The habit is always the impeding factor, and unless it is broken the prescribed treatment will be useless.

This leads us to consider the psycho-physical activities within the organism of which so-called habit is a manifestation. In a person with a satisfactory standard of co-ordination, moderation will be the rule. The reverse will be the case, to a greater or lesser degree, in the badly co-ordinated person; the habit of excess will gradually become more firmly established with too frequent repetition of the indulgence of the debauched sensory desires, thus making indulgence the rule and not the exception.

Obviously there was a time, before the cultivation of the alcoholic habit, when this man did not over-indulge in drinking. However, the reasons for beginning the habit of drinking too much would not help us very much, even if we could be certain of them. The important point to remember is that his sensory appreciation was unreliable and perverted, and he was in a state of psycho-physical malcoordination, so that he gradually became dominated by that sensory debauchery caused by excessive alcohol and other indulgences, and by the depressing and enervating conditions which ensue. These latter conditions are the most potent stimuli which make for *repetition of the habit at more and more frequent intervals.* The frequent repetition counteracts the depressing and enervating conditions for a time, so that, unfortunately, the process "makes the food it feeds on." Sensory debauchery increases rapidly until the functioning of the organism becomes utterly demoralized.

It is almost certain that, when he started drinking, this man was unaware of his lack of satisfactory co-ordination and sensory appreciation. He had simply taken alcohol occasionally, never meaning it to become a habit—or even suspecting that he lacked the ability either to continue drinking it only occasionally, or to stop altogether if he wished. This reveals the degree to which egotism may be subconsciously developed in the human creature, until it becomes a powerful factor in influencing the processes associated with subconscious and unreasoned conclusions. If he had consciously thought the matter out, he would have realized that his general standard of functioning and sensory appreciation were unsatisfactory, and that somehow he would have to make certain that they became satisfactory *before he allowed himself to entertain even mildly egotistical conclusions regarding his ability to fight his bad habits.* In other words, he would have realized *that in the matter of breaking a habit, the standard of sensory appreciation is the all-important factor.* His increasing desire for alcohol probably came very gradually, as did the corresponding decline in his co-ordination and sensory appreciation. Thus the abnormal desire would soon dominate the psycho-physical processes which could otherwise have been used in reasoning and common sense.

In all such experiences the person concerned is eventually forced to recognize the harmful effects of his or her habit, and then makes an effort to fight the desire and to eradicate the habit. But the effort is too often a feeble one, or is made along impossible lines. Some well-meaning friend may urge the person to use "willpower" to control the desire, *but the desire is a sensory desire, and the processes called "will-power" have long since been dominated by debauched sensory appreciation.* Salvation, therefore, lies in the restoration of a satisfactory, healthy sensory appreciation. In *Man's Supreme Inheritance,* I referred to that degenerate state where an organism desires sensory satisfaction through actual pain. In alcoholic excesses, each indulgence is followed by suffering, but even this does not act as a deterrent. We must, therefore, realize the enormous influence of perverted sensory desire on the human creature, and recognize that satisfactory development of control of the organism is impossible without that reliable sensory appreciation which goes hand in hand with normal sensory desires.

One more point. Fundamental desires and needs must be satisfied. If they are not, serious results must follow sooner or later. The fact that the attempt to satisfy needs leads many individuals to indulge in abuse and excess does not affect this conclusion. Abuse and excess are always associated with abnormality, and abnormality is due to abnormal conditions in the psycho-physical functioning of the organism. Abuse or excess is an attempt to satisfy a need which, originally normal, has become abnormal. As long as this abnormal need remains, it is useless to deny someone the means of indulging in abuse or excess. Instead, we should attempt to eradicate the abnormal conditions responsible for the excess and abuse, and so to restore normal functioning and reliable sensory appreciation.

Chapter 7

PSYCHO-PHYSICAL EQUILIBRIUM

The lack of satisfactory psycho-physical equilibrium in all human activities is one of the most striking manifestations of an imperfect functioning of the organism. The present subconscious faulty use of the mechanism in educational and other spheres makes for a gradual increase of this defective equilibrium. This is generally taken for granted—we expect defective equilibrium at a certain age, just as we expect the development of a flabby and protruding abdomen. Our contention that practice makes perfect is thereby shown to be misleading. And it also shows that there must be something wrong with our practice in the act of walking.

People walk without any clear understanding of the guiding principles which command the co-ordination and adjustment of the organism in the act of walking. When, therefore, a defect appears in the functioning of the organism, even though the person may be aware of the cause, they are unable to re-establish that standard of reliable sensory appreciation which would make it possible for them to eradicate the defect. Re-education on a general basis then becomes necessary to ensure a continued raising of the standard of psycho-physical equilibrium right on through life.

I will now endeavour to show that almost every attempt to

correct some supposed or real defect sets up the conditions for new defects to be developed which tend to further lower the standard of equilibrium. As this unsatisfactory condition develops, it unfortunately goes hand in hand with the desire to hurry too much, which is a subconscious endeavour to compensate for the growing lack of control. In extreme cases this manifestation is very pronounced. The person becomes conscious, first, of a difficulty which affects equilibrium in walking, and, without any attempt to discover the cause of the difficulty, he *tries* to "walk properly" — i.e., without the slight unsteadiness of which he is conscious. But the fact that this difficulty has developed is proof that this man's guiding sensations and general co-ordination are defective. Obviously, then, any subconscious effort on his part to "walk properly" will be carried out using the same faulty guiding sensations, and cannot therefore succeed.

During his "trial and error" experiences, his fear reflexes are being unduly excited by the fear of falling and by the general unreliability and uncertainty of the psycho-physical processes being used during these subconscious efforts. Taking the process as a whole, we will find that harmful psycho-physical conditions will be developed, which soon show themselves in other activities, and very often culminate in some serious crisis.

It is easy to trace the development of this lack of equilibrium in what is usually considered the "purely physical" sphere. Take the case of a boy who would be classed as a "good walker." Let us assume he is injured in a fall at the age of thirteen, confined to bed and treated by a doctor. The cessation of activities produces a generally weakened condition and also specific difficulties with the injured part of the organism. The result is that at the psychological moment when the boy makes his first attempt to resume walking, certain factors will impede him. He will immediately attempt to overcome them by "trying to walk properly" as he understands it. These attempts will be on a subconscious plan of "trial and error" because it is almost certain that he has never known *how* he walked, never had the least idea of it.

(Note: The reader probably knows of such a case where the person is now walking about to his or her own satisfaction. However, my point is, that the person is not capable of judging whether their use of their psycho-physical mechanisms in walking is satisfactory or not. Anyone with expert knowledge in this field could point to certain harmful defects in the person's use which are the combined result of the injury, the various experiences in treatment and recovery, and the attempts "to walk," all of which show a comparative weakness and an interference with equilibrium and control.)

It is necessary to analyze the psycho-physical processes involved in the boy's efforts to walk, because success in such efforts demands a high standard of co-ordinated functioning of the organism. This is not at the command of a person who has had such an injury and who has experienced the subsequent treatment and gradual recovery. Real success is practically impossible for the following reasons.

The boy's attempts to walk would be made at a time when he was conscious of a general weakness in his organism, a comparative loss of control, a lack of confidence, and a whole series of hopes and fears about what he will or will not be able to do. These are fears which result from the painful incorrect subconscious attempts to use the parts of the organism which have been injured. This whole combination of psycho-physical conditions constitutes a set of experiences which are different from those which existed before the accident. Each subconscious attempt to walk brings awareness of shortcomings, of strange, alarming sensations, and increases the real difficulties, that is, those concerned with the correct psycho-physical use on which "walking properly" depends.

Thus the attempt to walk properly by subconscious guidance is simply an attempt to revert to the same habits established in the act of walking before his accident: to an instinctive way of walking. If the conditions for the instinctive behavior are changed quickly, as in such an accident, then there will be an interference with the reliability of the working of that instinct.

This illustration provides us with a splendid instance of a definite need calling for new experiences in psycho-physical use. The boy wishes to walk. The stimulus produces a response involving subconscious guidance and control which is habitual and which depends for efficiency on a given standard of co-ordinated functioning of the organism. Unfortunately, this standard has been lowered by his experiences associated with the accident and his psycho-physical machinery does not work as well as before. He is aware of this fact. This causes him to "try harder," but, working on a subconscious basis, he has no alternative but to continue the unintelligent method of "trial and error."

In a procedure founded on the principles of re-education on a conscious general basis, the experiences of the boy would have differed as follows. In the first place, we would not allow the boy to try to "walk properly" until he has been given, by expert manipulation, correct experiences in the general use of the mechanism and has become well acquainted with the correct guiding and controlling directions which would assist in the securing of the *means* he should use the mechanism in the act of walking.

We advocate that the boy be taught to stop trying to improve his walking. The peculiarities in the boy's psycho-physical use of his organism as a whole are noted and the teacher would endeavour to convince him by demonstration that his efforts to "muddle through by instinct" are not only futile but quite absurd. The teacher also shows him that, as soon as he receives the stimulus to walk, he must inhibit his desire to do so, in order to prevent the wrong subconscious use of the mechanism associated with his conception of "walking." It is explained to him that it is his habitual use in walking, associated with unreliable sensory appreciation, which has caused the faulty use of his mechanisms, resulting in the weakness and difficulty with which we are contending.

When the boy is familiar with the use of inhibition, he is shown how to employ the new guiding directions which, with the help of expert manipulation, will bring about the satisfactory use of the mechanism in a sitting, prone, or other position. These experiences must be repeated until the new, reliable sensory appreciation becomes established. Eventually, a change will take place in the use of the psycho-physical mechanisms in general, which will bring about satisfactory co-ordination and adjustment. This improvement is brought about consciously by the boy and ensures a corresponding improvement in his walking.

The reader must understand that the details involved in this process cannot be listed here, as all individuals are different. The teacher's aim is to cause the pupil to be conscious of what he should or should *not* do, and to teach him to apply conscious control not only in walking, but in all the acts of daily life. The pupil, therefore, is not taught to perform certain new exercises or to assume new postures for a given time each day. He is shown *how* he may check the faulty use of his mechanisms in everyday life.

An increase in lack of equilibrium in the so-called "physical" sphere will be found to have a corresponding lack of equilibrium in so-called "mental" spheres. In any consideration of "mental" and "physical" phenomena it must be remembered that in our present stage of evolution on the subconscious plane, the response to any stimulus is at least—probably more than—75% subconscious response (mainly feeling) as against 25% any other response.

When these facts are fully realized by all those interested in education and in the conduct of life generally, there may be some chance of the realization of those commendable ideals so many of us have for the uplifting of humankind.

PART 3

SENSORY APPRECIATION IN ITS RELATION TO HUMANITY'S NEEDS

Chapter 1

"KNOWING ONESELF"

Those who give thought to the present trend of human endeavour in political, social, industrial, and other spheres will recognize that our times are "out of joint." Many will admit that the majority of people are out of communication with their reasoning. People are struggling blindly for their individual betterment, without any clear understanding of the causes of their difficulties, or of the fundamental principles which constitute in application the satisfactory *means* of preventing or overcoming these difficulties.

"Man know thyself" is an old axiom, but in my opinion the more fundamental one is "Man know your needs." We have seen that reliable sensory appreciation is essential to that co-ordinated psycho-physical growth and development of the individual which is, in turn, fundamental to the satisfactory growth and development of the mass. In order to ensure this, it is essential to command the "means" of recognizing and supplying the real needs of the individual.

Unfortunately, our attempts to supply and satisfy these needs in the educational, social, political, industrial, religious, and other spheres, have proved more or less of a failure up to now. This is largely because our efforts on a subconscious basis have been directed mainly to evolving methods of teaching, treatment, conduct, guidance, and control to meet the demands of the mass, instead of making the primary application of the principles involved an individual one on a conscious basis. The foregoing leads us to consider the relative possibilities of plans for human development on both the conscious and subconscious planes.

On the subconscious plane, the orthodox plan has been, and still is, to eradicate "physical" defects by means of physical culture, exercises, etc., and "mental" shortcomings by different forms of "mental" training: specific systems for developing memory, and so on. The deductions leading to the adoption of such methods were based on wrong premises because the fundamental principle of conscious control was ignored. When "physical" and "mental" methods are employed separately, any apparent improvement will only be a specific one and will go on to cultivate harmful defects of which the teacher and pupil are at first ignorant. Sooner or later they reveal themselves and gradually become established as habits.

The progress made in recent years in "psychological" knowledge leaves no doubt that human beings are too often unaware of their most striking psycho-physical defects. Before we can make any real attempt to reach a satisfactory state of awareness with regard to self-knowledge, we must cultivate an increasing use of reasoning in conscious endeavour and, when we reach a satisfactory standard of readjustment and co-ordination through new and reliable sensory appreciation, we must put this conscious use of the self into practice, in every act of daily life.

"Knowing oneself" is part and parcel of the process so that our degree of self-knowledge will increase and keep pace with our development in conscious psycho-physical control. This knowledge should be the foundation of the act of living in all spheres, and will be so when the education and general development of children are built on the principles of constructive, conscious control. On this principle we can continue to raise the standard of self-knowledge and thus of everything else we know in all spheres of learning.

A friend of mine who wanted to impress me with his knowledge of up-to-date psychology, admitted that he based what he knew on his study of human history as written by eminent historians. I could not bring myself to disillusion him by suggesting that the real history of human endeavour, as a guide to up-to-date psychology, has not been written by the historians—that it has, in fact, yet to be set down.

By human endeavour, I mean individual human endeavour in connection with individual development and growth. We must, therefore, eliminate the record of humanity's activities in wars, and other spheres in which it is swayed chiefly by the herd instinct, from any real history of human endeavour. Activities where the command or example of one person is immediately followed by the rest as an unthinking, unintelligent, automatic mass as in wars, may, I admit, be of great interest to many people; but it is of infinitesimal value, particularly where humanity's future is concerned, when compared with the individual effort of the human being struggling daily to find a solution to the flesh-and-blood difficulties which directly concern his or her well-being. I refer to difficulties which confront us in our attempts to adapt to ever-changing conditions as we evolve from the uncivilized to the civilized state.

This is equally true of the everyday development of the ordinary person in all areas of human activity, because we are beset with contending and disorganizing forces in the working of the psycho-physical organism of each individual, as we rapidly develop "mental" processes at an ever-increasing pace. At the same time we are attempting to employ the so-called physical processes which for years have become less and less satisfactorily controlled and directed. This has resulted in the lowering of the standard of psycho-physical equilibrium and co-ordination.

The long line of daily difficulties which we now face is equaled only by the series of shattered hopes that have followed each subconsciously directed, specific "end-gaining" attempt to solve these difficulties. Each failure makes "the food it feeds on," and the "trial and error" method has been persistently adhered to despite the fact of its unreliability.

I will now deal from this point of view with certain systems of education and development which have public attention at the moment, and which were designed to meet certain difficulties and defects. I will show that the hopes of those concerned cannot be justified, because these systems were conceived on a specific basis and rely on subconscious experience. We have reached a stage in our evolution when we should refuse to consider any new system of education or development which is not built on a conscious basis.

One such system in England and America simply uses the same principles which were used by circus trainers in our grandfathers' time in training horses to perform certain steps to music, etc. It can be dismissed without further comment.

Another system which is considered to be progressive attempts to improve children's senses of sight, feeling, taste, hearing, touch, and so on by using an organized series of materials and educative toys. This aims once again at a *specific* and not a *general* development—a fatal mistake when we consider the interdependence of what has been separated into "mental" and "physical" in the human organism. It is quite possible that a child, by using this material, may gain a certain facility in the use of his or her hands, or a specific development, say, of the sense of touch. But if the child, in making the movements necessary for a particular occupation, is relying on imperfect sensory appreciation in the general use of his or her organism, it must follow that any specific improvement will be accompanied by a use of mechanisms, which, faulty to start with, will become steadily more faulty the harder the child tries, or the more absorbed the child becomes in working subconsciously for his or her end. Specific improvement may happen, but only at the expense of good general use of the organism. In my experience, children who have had specialized training in their early years, have more than the usual number of psycho-physical defects. Their sensory appreciation is more than usually unreliable, and my argument is that this must be so where any specific development is sought on a subconscious basis.

The interdependence of the "mental" and the "physical" and of the muscular mechanism in general has long since been recognized in theory, but methods of education aiming at specific development remain in vogue. With regard to this specific development of a particular sense, it is now well known that the sense of sight, for instance, is greatly affected by the "muscle-pulls" of the organism in general and this applies to the other senses also. For many years, we have had practical proof of the improvement that can be effected in the sense of sight of pupils who have been re-educated on a general basis of conscious control. This improvement has always followed an improvement in the use of the whole organism.

This is the point which must always be emphasized by those who advocate re-education on a general basis. The person with defective sight will have a number of other psycho-physical defects, and re-education on a general basis must precede any attempt at specific re-education.

If children were re-educated using conscious control, 75% of the ordinary sense imperfections and difficulties with technique would never be encountered by the teachers working in educational and other spheres. It does not require any special degree of intelligence to realize the tremendous amount of time and energy that would be saved if we adopted the comprehensive and constructive principles given here and applied them to all forms of human development in our efforts to ensure a progressive civilization.

The consciously co-ordinated child will possess a psycho-physical mechanism which will tend to function at its maximum in all activities according to the standard of co-ordination reached. The teacher can then draw from the child the very best that the particular psycho-physical organism can give, and can also be confident of increasing improvement, without the undue excitement of the fear reflexes and without undue effort.

Think, on the other hand, of the harmful psycho-physical effect on a child beset with all the impeding factors resulting from a condition of poor co-ordination, if, when learning for instance to write, he takes up the pencil for the first time and holds it with strained and cramped fingers caused by stress and strain in the organism in general. Even if the teacher does not tell the child directly that his use of the pencil is not what it should be, the child will probably be aware of a lack of control. Sooner or later, the teacher will try and improve the child's writing, and may succeed up to a point; but it will be a very poor result compared to the standard that would be attained if the child were first re-educated and re-adjusted on a general basis.

As I have already stated, with the usual education on a specific basis, we are repeatedly confronted with new and increasing difficulties calling for eradication—difficulties which we have actually cultivated ourselves. The efforts made in education to counteract, by specific means, the retarding influences of certain defects over-look the fact that they have been developed or further complicated by this same educational process.

The process becomes operative as soon as the child goes to school. Experiences gained in school too often lead to such complications if from the beginning the child is functioning nearer to its minimum than to its maximum. Most of these defects, however, would not have occurred, if the child's psycho-physical functioning had been satisfactory on starting school. The establishment of satisfactory psycho-physical functioning should therefore be the first consideration in any sound educational plan. To attempt to educate an imperfectly co-ordinated child on a specific basis is an unreasoning process, especially when we consider the important part played in the child's life by the process of imitation.

Chapter 2

IMITATION

The psycho-physical process called *imitation* operates in most people to a high degree compared with other fundamental processes. We are all aware of this aptitude. Subconscious imitation of the characteristics of others is a factor which plays a great part in our development and growth, as well as in our use of our psycho-

physical selves. Overwhelming proof of this natural ⸱
the harmful consequences which can result from it is a
us look at some of the chief factors responsible for the d⸱
ing results accrued from imitation in civilization.

This book deals with the defects, peculiarities, imperfect ⸱
and so on in the human organism of the majority of people. ⸱
contends that, in some, these shortcomings are so extreme that
they could be considered to constitute a form of deformity. Herein
lies the cause of the harmful results of imitation, because the process remains inoperative unless there is something striking to
imitate. The chief stimulus to imitation comes from our perception, subconscious or conscious, of some characteristic or striking
feature of another person—and these manifestations are usually
psycho-physical peculiarities. In all areas of everyday life, the dangers from the individual imitation of others' defects are very great.
It is, therefore, of the utmost importance that these dangers be
eliminated, or at least minimized, in our learning—particularly
where there is a teacher-pupil relationship such as in schools, or
any other situation of close contact which makes imitation possible.

As we have seen, most children at school manifest shortcomings in the use of themselves and all kinds of drills and exercises
are used to attempt to eradicate them. Yet, except in very rare instances, the teachers themselves are beset with exaggerated forms
of such defects. If teachers are worthy of the name, it is certain that
their pupils will be influenced by them in many ways, and that
pupils will tend subconsciously to imitate them. The most striking
characteristics of the teacher are the most powerful stimuli for this
imitation. Peculiarities in the quality of voice, for example, or the
manner of opening the mouth, of using the arms, of defective
speech, of standing, walking, sitting, etc. All this has serious consequences because the imitation of the teachers' own unreliable
sensory appreciation and use of the organism becomes an impeding factor for the pupils.

In any sphere of subconscious learning, the teacher and the

_wrong idea that the pupil, by observing the teacher
_thing successfully, will be able to copy it and succeed
_pupil is convinced of this and the teacher, too, is certain
_he teaches the pupil to do as he believes he does himself, he
_enable the pupil to succeed.

(Note: Take, for example, a singer who is forced to retire from public performance because of throat trouble and becomes a teacher. I recall hearing two such singers performing, and knew they would be forced to retire soon, because no human throat and accessories could withstand indefinitely the abuse they suffered in the way of strain, larynx displacement, and chest and abdominal distortion. When they took up teaching, the misuse of their psycho-physical mechanisms in singing was imparted to their pupils, that is, the methods of singing and breathing which they believed in. They believed their methods were correct ones, because they had used them during their own time of learning, and had practiced them right up until they began teaching. The fact that these very methods had caused them to lose their voices did not even occur to them, or would they be teaching the same techniques to others? The power of the human being to hypnotize oneself is nowhere more apparent than in such instances of human idiosyncrasy as this.)

If a pupil of an art form is sent to watch a great artist at work, the pupil is almost invariably more impressed by some characteristic of the artist than he or she is by the artist's "better parts."

The characteristics of the artist are seized on by the pupil as factors essential to the pupil's own improvement, but experience constantly proves this to be a mistaken belief. In the first place, the characteristics may be faults which the genius of the particular artist enables him or her to defy. And secondly, it is possible that the artist succeeds _in spite of them, rather than because of them._

(Note: Unfortunately, this tendency exists in all spheres of learning. Take sport for instance: Smith used a crouch and whirlwind drive; Gose was noted for his forehand drive;

Doherty for an unchanged grip, and so on. Other player.
imitated these things in the hope of improving their own
game, but experience has constantly proved this a mistaken
idea for the reasons given above.)

But even if the characteristics of the artist noted by the pupil
were of value, the only way the pupil could make practical use of
them would be by a careful study of the artist's general use, of
which the characteristics are but special manifestations. The pupil
would need re-education to be able to command the same general
use of the organism, to the standard of the expert the pupil wants
to imitate.

Chapter 3

CONCENTRATION AND THE SUSTAINED (CONTINUOUS) PROJECTION OF DIRECTIONS

The experiences outlined in connection with imitation reveal that
this conception involves specific attempts to gain an "end." In
other words, *specifics* are selected for *specific* imitation. So the
process of imitation becomes one of "fixating on specific points or
objects," that is, of what is known as "concentration."

The conception of concentration is a disastrous and narrowing
one. When a person tries to concentrate, harmful manifestations
become more and more exaggerated according to the degree with
which the teacher urges the pupil to develop this doubtful acquisition.

Where did this idea of "concentration" come from? At what
stage in the process of education was it considered necessary?

There can be little doubt that the conception and use of

...centration sprang from a desire to have the same ease, spontaneity, and healthy enjoyment of the organism considered successful and which is characteristic of people who are said to "give their attention" to whatever they wish to do. What has not been realized, however, is that it is only those children with imperfect psychophysical functioning who show symptoms of "mind-wandering," lack of spontaneity of observation and of curiosity, etc.—granted, of course, a reasonable approach by the teacher. The child of two hundred years ago was born with comparatively reliable instincts, adequate respiratory need, and the psycho-physical equipment which would have allowed satisfactory development if his education had been based on a principle of conscious control and of the co-ordinated "means." Unfortunately, it was not, but was worked out on a subconscious end-gaining basis and the harmful effects of this grew very rapidly until the child developed an inability to pay attention, that is, began to "mind-wander." When the teachers in authority recognized that this "mind-wandering" required a remedy, what else could they do, subconsciously directed as they themselves were, but adopt a system which would attempt to "hold the mind" (attention) to one subject?

(Note: The recognition of the defect of "mind-wandering" and the remedy adopted for it has its parallel in the first recognition of "physical" deterioration and the remedy applied. The false principle underlying both remedies is the same.)

The word "concentrate" is defined as "to force or cause to move to a common center; to bring to bear on one object," the latter being the general acceptance of the word.

Here, then, was the remedy which has now been applied for many many years and which has today become a universal belief in what is conceived of as "concentration." You will not find a person who does not believe in concentration. Tell a friend, for the sake of argument, that you do not believe in concentration but think that it has harmful effects and you will almost certainly hear remarks like, "But surely we should concentrate our minds on what we are doing?" and "One is naturally anxious to do one's best and surely

the degree of success depends on one's power of concentration."
And so on.

Again, people say they can only work successfully if they have
perfect quiet, that any interruption breaks the train of thought,
and many other points will be brought forward to support their
belief in concentration. There is only one satisfactory way to end
such arguments as this: by means of practical demonstration. A
teacher of conscious control is prepared to convince anyone who
can and will trust his or her eyes in such a demonstration. Statements and arguments in connection with psycho-physical activities should not be accepted unless the person making them can
give a practical demonstration of their truth, while showing, at the
same time, that they themselves are in communication with their
reasoning. By way of proof then, observe the psycho-physical
manifestations of the person who believes in concentration during
reading, writing, thinking, or any other daily activity. Observe the
strained expression of the eyes, an expression of anxiety and un-
easiness denoting unduly excited fear reflexes; in some cases the
eyes may be distorted and the whole expression one that is recognized as the self-hypnotic stare. Observe also the harmful degree of
tension throughout the whole organism. This could not be otherwise, because the person, instead of reasoning out the cause of his
or her defects, is subconsciously *trying* (by "trial and error") to
overpower one set of so-called "mental" projections and "physical"
tensions by a still more powerful set.

Consider the example of the act of sitting in a chair. The pupil
does this habitually with a great deal of unnecessary tension.
Suppose the teacher points this out and reasons out with him or
her the means of performing this act without strain. The teacher
gives the pupil the necessary directions and the reliable sensory
appreciation required for the satisfactory carrying-out of these
directions. Suppose further that the pupil, instead of carrying
out the instructions from the teacher in the order given, starts to
"concentrate" on them. What will she really be doing? In a specific
way, she will be concentrating on one direction and comparatively

neglecting the others, while in a general way, she will be overpowering the new conscious directions, by a still more powerful set of orders which are in accordance with her conception of *the act of concentration.* This is an unreasoned procedure and all that she accomplishes is the reinforcement of all the old misdirected, subconscious activity connected with the act of sitting down. She sets up a civil war in the organism.

The point is made even more clearly when a pupil is asked to sit quietly and do nothing while the teacher moves some part of his body for him. In my experience, as soon as the pupil is asked not to do anything, he immediately shows all those signs of fixity and strain which he associates with actually doing something, that is, he concentrates. Point this out and he will protest, "I am trying to do nothing!" He actually believes he has something *to do* to do nothing. We are led to such a point by our belief in concentration!

This whole matter shows the danger of applying a specific remedy to a psycho-physical defect like "mind-wandering," which has its basis in an imperfect use of the psycho-physical mechanism in general. When a person develops "mind-wandering," there is a condition of unreliable sensory appreciation and undue stress and strain during activities which is always associated with imperfect co-ordination. To anyone in this condition any specific remedy is fraught with danger. With conscious control such dangers can be escaped, but almost never on a subconscious basis.

As to the narrowing effect of "concentration": It is difficult to find an adult who can think of more than one thing at a time, or use simultaneously even two parts of the body in a co-ordinated manner. Co-ordinated use of different parts of the mechanism calls for the continuous projection of directions to these parts, the primary direction being *continued,* while the others connected with the secondary part of the movement are projected, and so on. Ordinarily, in attempts to use two or more parts, the primary direction is *immediately* forgotten as soon as the person starts to move. This applies to all other directions concerning other parts of the movement, and is another example of concentrated effort on the "end-gaining" principle. The *continuous* projection of directions, on the other hand calls for a broad, reasoning attitude, so that the pupil has not only a clear conception of the directions essential (the means) for the correct performance of a movement, but can also project these directions in their right relationship to one another, the co-ordinated series of orders resulting in a co-ordinated use of the organism.

Imperfect co-ordination, then, involves reliance on the "end-gaining" principle. It is therefore not surprising that so many pupils have the habit of projecting unconsidered and *disconnected* directions. This means that the directions have not been reasoned out with regard to the co-ordinated use of the parts concerned and *this results in a malcoordinated movement*. When, therefore, such a pupil comes for remedial work through conscious control and is asked to project his directions continuously, he naturally finds great difficulty in breaking his habit of discontinuous attention and haphazard, subconscious guidance and direction. As a rule, the pupil has no conception of linking up the different parts of the movement and the related directions. She believes that she cannot "bring her mind to bear" on more than one point at a time. This is entirely in line with the definition of concentration given above, but it is a delusion on the pupil's part, because she has been "bringing her mind to bear" on several things at once *subconsciously* all her life, or she would not be able to carry out the simplest of her daily activities.

An illustration will make this clear. A person rises from a chair to speak to a friend who comes into the room. The stimulus to rise comes to him and his response to this is his decision to stand up. As soon as the decision is made, the messages connected with the well-established habit of rising from sitting to standing are sent to the psycho-physical mechanisms involved, and the act of rising occurs. The person immediately engages in a conversation for half an hour. He is absorbed by the requirements of the discussion and will tell you that he must concentrate on what is being said in order to do his best. The point of interest for us is the consider-

ation of the *means* by which he remains standing *of which he is
not and never has been conscious.* The messages sent after his
decision to stand up must be maintained until he decides to adopt
some other position. It will be clear, therefore, that the human
being has developed the ability to sustain continuous subconscious
directions to himself. Insistence, then, on the necessity and importance of sustained directions in the work of re-education is based,
not on a new, but on a very old and fundamental principle in human development.

To repeat: The prevalent belief in concentration goes hand in
hand with the acceptance of the "end-gaining" principle, rather
than the principle of thinking out clearly and *connectedly* the
means of securing an end, and of "bringing the mind to bear" on
as many subjects (continuous directions) as is necessary for the
purpose and which converge to a common consequence. In concentration the person deliberately develops the practice of focusing
the mind on one subject only.

In the acts of everyday life, it will be found that in the opinion
of ninety-nine people out of a hundred, the consideration of the
"means" of using the psycho-physical organism would be a hin-
drance or an interference. These people are confident that they
cannot attend to more than one thing at a time. It never occurs to
them that the psycho-physical self is the instrument by which they
carry out their daily business, that their standard of success depends on the standard of functioning of this instrument, and that
it is therefore essential to pay attention to this wonderful machine
if success in any business or profession is desired. The confession
that they are incapable of carrying on these two all important and
interdependent psycho-physical processes simultaneously is tanta-
mount to admitting that if they give due attention to the *means* of
gaining their "end" they will be unable to attend to the "end,"
which is absurd! Such a confession illustrates the stage where
humankind, as a mass, is today on the evolutionary plane. It
certainly is not a very high stage, considering the human

creature's potentialities and the fact that, in the development of the animal and the primitive person, the two processes (mental and physical) concerned with use of the creature's self in everyday life were interdependent.

In a society which believes in and practices "concentration," the individual person's conception of what exactly "concentration" is will be in accordance with his psycho-physical defects; and if he becomes aware of these defects, he believes that what he understands to be "concentration" will remove them. Once he has adopted this narrowing process, it is not surprising that he finds it impossible to do or think of more than one thing at a time. The harmful psycho-physical condition thus established does not make for a satisfactory condition of all-round functioning.

On the other hand, in watching the progress of people who are re-educated on a general basis, we see that it is possible to learn to give continuous attention to the *means* of using the mechanism throughout daily life. The human organism is capable of doing many things at the same time, and, in those cases where a unified psycho-physical co-ordination is operative (true concentration), the person is as unaware of the operation of concentration as she is of the process of co-ordination. As a matter of fact, it is unlikely that such a person will have given thought to the necessity for concentration; she will not have recognized the need for it or have considered it a process requiring special attention.

The satisfactory conditions in the co ordinated person represent a form of concentration which cannot be secured by "thinking of concentration" or by telling another to think of it. This whole book is devoted to exposing the fallacy of asking any imperfectly co-ordinated person to attempt to eradicate his or her defects by some written or spoken instructions. It is certain that any person who is unable to concentrate, in the sense of giving due attention to the matter in hand, is an imperfectly co-ordinated person. To ask such a person to overcome the failure to concentrate by "concentrating" in accordance with their conception of these acts, is to cause a harmful and artificial division of the personality. What is needed is the restoration of a satisfactory condition of psycho-physical co-ordination on a general basis, which involves the use of the true processes of concentration.

Chapter 4

MEMORY AND FEELING

As we have seen, most teachers of today are disturbed by children's growing lack of attention in school. The children, as they say, "cannot concentrate." They do not, however, seem to be equally disturbed by the increase in what is called "loss of memory." Indeed, they are as yet unaware of the fact that the psycho-physical efforts made in learning to "concentrate" tend to interfere with the processes of remembering (in its broadest sense), with the result that unequal, narrowing, and often inadequate impressions are registered.

Many people acknowledge their growing "loss of memory," and various systems of "mental training" are used in an attempt to improve this situation. Here again, it is of interest for us that all these systems are based on "end-gaining" principles and, as in the case of "mind-wandering," no attempt is made to associate the problem of "bad memory" with other psycho-physical defects.

At a stage in our development when "loss of memory" has become more or less a general defect, we must consider the psycho-physical conditions involved, as well as the various imperfect uses of the psycho-physical mechanisms which cause the development of these conditions.

Memory is the impression which is registered as the result of some stimulus. The lasting quality of the impression depends on certain psycho-physical processes concerned with the registering of the impressions. The effectiveness of these processes depends, in turn, on the general psycho-physical condition and especially on the standard of sensory appreciation. Environment also influences these conditions at the moment of registration of the impression; yet a further factor is the individual's ability to link up the knowledge or the experience given by any stimulus with the knowledge and experiences already acquired. As we are aware, our habits of life are the manifestations of our psycho-physical functioning. This functioning governs our habits in registering impressions in connection with memory, just as it influences all our other activities.

There can be little doubt that the growing habit of the reading of newspapers and light literature rather than written matter which is to be retained as valuable knowledge, has been accompanied by harmful psycho-physical habits, which today are seriously affecting the human memory. People study and memorize printed matter because they hope by this means to acquire lasting knowledge. As a rule, they read newspapers, magazines, etc., hastily, without attempting to memorize them. Similarly, they simply glance at the news of the day and register only the faintest impression. This probably serves them for that day or week, but in a month's time they will be hazy about it, and in a year's time the impression may be completely effaced. Thus, millions of people "skim" over books, receiving only faint impressions. This is a harmful habit which rapidly becomes established, and very soon the person becomes aware of a growing loss of memory in all spheres.

This increase in our "loss of memory," more pronounced over the last twenty or thirty years, must be checked or it will undermine the usefulness of our psycho-physical processes. For reasoning is dependent on the association of remembered facts with other facts, which are stimuli to the processes concerned. When the memory fails, therefore, the ability to reason satisfactorily is suspended.

It will be useful to consider the interdependence and the action of sensory appreciation and so-called "mental" activity before going on to deal with the effects of certain sensory habits concerned with memory. The idea conveyed by the voice of one person reaches the consciousness of another through hearing; the written word through sight; other stimuli are received through touch, taste, smell, etc. In a general way, our senses play the leading part in the processes of remembering and reasoning—in fact, they do so in all psycho-physical activity. The standard of functioning of these processes depends, therefore, directly or indirectly, on the standard of sensory appreciation.

Readers may give examples of remarkable feats of memory by people in specific spheres, but my experience of these cases is that excellence in one sphere will be equaled by a lack of it in all others. These cases are simply abnormal.

Here is an interesting instance of a young man who could memorize train time-tables with only a cursory glance at each page. Three months later, he could still tell you the time of any train on that list. But the same man would often leave his umbrella on the bus, or go out to buy some domestic article and return home without it. In fact, in general, judged by the ordinary standard of human intelligence, he was quite a hopeless person. This man is a fine example of a remarkable feat of memory in a specific sphere, accompanied by defective remembering and reasoning in general activity, associated with delusive sensory appreciation.

(Note: We must beware of placing exaggerated value on intelligence in some specific sphere. Judgment must always be made of the person's intelligent activities on a general basis, in the process of living and all-round usefulness. The genuine specialist must always primarily be a proficient general practitioner in his trade, profession or other activities. Satisfactory growth as a specialist demands a continuous development of those experiences which only the general practitioner can command. This matter of correct relative values is of the utmost importance since if we are to establish a sound basis for judgment in the future, we must first give consideration to the *means* of carrying out any act rather than to the act itself. What useful part does the performance of an act play in a person's so-called "intellectual" or "physical" development, if the person is harmed by the process?)

There is little doubt that most of the early bad habits which result in "loss of memory" are actually cultivated during the different processes in all forms of education. This cultivation is most pronounced when the pupil is taught to perform some "physical" act. Therefore, now that we have been unreasoning enough to force every unfortunate school child, irrespective of his or her individual standard of sensory appreciation, to learn "physical" drill or to perform exercises, we must expect a more rapid development of "loss of memory" than during previous years in the majority of people.

If one observes carefully any sports lesson in school, one will see that the children are trying to carry out the teacher's instructions by "physically" performing some small part of the instructions which has specifically appealed to each of them. They are so absorbed in this part of the performance that they are oblivious to any other part of the instructions given by the teacher. If the teacher questions the pupil he or she will find that this is true. An expert in psycho-physical re-education has only to observe the expression in the pupil's eyes, and certain other manifestations, to be quite certain.

A recent experience I had during a lesson demonstrates this. I asked my pupil to listen to my instructions regarding the use of the lips, tongue, and jaw in that order. (This pupil had, of course, already been given the necessary work in connection with the general co-ordinated use of the mechanism.) The first time the instructions were given it was obvious that the pupil was attempting to memorize them as they were spoken by trying to "feel" them rather than acquiring the instructions by "committing them to memory."

The pupil was asked to listen a second time and was asked not to try to move the parts concerned, but merely to listen and re-member. Before the teacher could finish giving the instructions, however, the pupil was again making movements with his lips, tongue, and jaw. He was asked why he was making these move-ments. He replied "I am trying to make certain of the instructions." It was explained to him that his method was not a satisfactory method, and that, instead, what he needed to do was to memorize the instructions first before attempting to carry them out, and that only when the correct *means* were included in the instructions would there be any chance of his carrying them out successfully.

In his attempts, therefore, to memorize the instructions, the pupil was following a preconceived plan. The act of memorizing, in his conception, was much more a "physical" than a "mental" act, and if his psycho-physical functioning had been up to a reliable standard, the plan may have proved successful. Now comes the most interesting part. The following morning he was asked to re-peat the instructions but could not recall them. His plan of memo-rizing the instructions by trying to feel them had failed because of his imperfect sensory appreciation. The habit of attempting to per-form an act before the guiding directions concerned have been memorized is associated with an inadequate use of inhibition com-pared with volition. Thus, when the pupil faces a new experience, his inhibitory processes are ineffective. This means that he is gradually cultivating an unbalanced psycho-physical condition in which the "mental" impressions he receives when learning some-thing are unduly faint and unreliable.

In order to restore balance, it is necessary first to develop a con-scious, reasoning inhibition (prevention). The person must learn to say "No" to every stimulus to psycho-physical activity until hav-ing taken time to consider what are the reasonable *means* of achieving any end. He or she must then repeat and memorize the directions relative to those means before using them in guiding the mechanisms essential to the particular psycho-physical act to be performed.

(Note: We have recently seen the rise and fall of a system

which claimed to restore failing memory and by specific means bestow "mental" blessings. These, however, were quite beyond the most sanguine expectations of any sane person who had even a reasonable knowledge of the fundamental psycho-physical processes essential to satisfactory memorizing. The rapid rise and fall of this system gives food for thought, especially because of the eulogies published about the system, some by people who are recognized as leaders of thought in our time. It is unfortunate that we cannot call these people to account and force them to justify these eulogies for a system which was, after all, just a piece of "mental gymnastics," totally ignoring the general psycho-physical conditions of the individual. The psycho-physical defects were the cause of the "mental" shortcomings, a cause of which these leaders of thought were totally ignorant. In the twentieth century, just as in the days of the cave-man, the blind continue to lead the blind, but the process brings more disastrous results nowadays than it could in those early days of humankind's more limited psycho-physical activities.)

Chapter 5

COMPLEXITY AND COMPLICATIONS IN RELATION TO STRESS AND STRAIN

We are frequently told that the cause of most of our difficulties is the increasing pace and complexity of the demands of modern day life. It is much more to the point to say that our real difficulties arise from the almost universal adoption of the "end-gaining" principle in our attempts to meet these demands. The result is that we cause ourselves much stress and strain, which, in our ignorance, we regard as something apart from ourselves. We make subconscious, unintelligent efforts to adapt ourselves to what we consider to be our "advancing" civilization.

First, we have stress and strain within ourselves—that is, in the functioning of the psycho-physical mechanisms as we use them to satisfy our needs in maintaining health and in general activity. Then we have the stress and strain of the "fight for life," "the complexity of life," and so on—in other words, the stress and strain occasioned by our efforts to make the wheels of the complex man-made machinery of life go round in social, industrial, political, religious, educational, and moral spheres.

These two areas of stress and strain are inseparable because our activities in all these spheres depend on the experiences of our individual psycho-physical life. The false "end-gaining" principles applied to living in both instances are entirely responsible for the unsettled, stressful state which prevails at this very moment. Had the prophets, philosophers, and leaders of the past recognized this fact, they would have shown proof of clear analysis and foresight. Unfortunately, the growing tendency towards disunion, dissatisfaction, enmity, and discord instead of unity, satisfaction, good-fellowship, and peace may be attributed to the unfortunate fact that they did not do so. We have unrest in people everywhere which is thought to be caused by "nerves" ["stress" —ed.] or some such symptom, and the alarming feature of it all is that it is an increasing unrest.

The venomous and penetrating roots of the cancer of disunion continue to spread and have caused deterioration and demoralization in the vital parts of our psycho-mechanical life as well as our social and industrial life, and the difficulties in applying the principles which make for unity are already alarming. It is universally contended that unity is needed ("united we stand, divided we fall") and this has a universal application to satisfactory human endeavour. Yet in almost every area of human activity we find this growing tendency to disunion.

Surely it is reasonable to conclude that the cause is due to some serious defect in the fundamentals of man-made institutions. If the principles involved had been sound, their application would have tended towards unity. We cannot fail to recognize that an alarming growth of disunion leading to complications in human activity is present here. If we keep to our current system of life, living will be still more complicated in one hundred years' time and so on, until it is so complicated that we shall not even have time to live!

The foregoing shows that the unreasoned processes which cause harmful complications in education are paramount in every other sphere of life. The parallel to the failure in our teaching methods is found in our efforts to progress in social, political, industrial, moral, and other spheres, where the "remedy" is often more harmful than the disease. How absurd, for instance, are the attempts for the "uplifting of man" in industry, when these are associated with that demoralizing conception which has led to the lowering of the standard of people's daily efforts to the level of the less capable and so to the lowering of the standard of individual psycho-physical functioning in the sphere of labor. We are all aware of the psycho-physical happiness gained from giving our best in our daily lives, and there is little hope for the person who is no longer able to gain satisfaction from this source.

Again, in politics, what could be more stupid than the ordinary party attitude, leading, as it does, to undesirable individual manifestations of deception, prejudice, egotism, and "emotional gusts"? It is unreasonable and dishonest to withhold support from or denounce measures which one believes to be right and of value to humanity, simply because they are put forward by the political party to which one does not belong. Under the present plan, politics and deception are interdependent. The politician seeking re-election will resort to forms of deception which he or she would not stoop to in other walks of life—particularly in making promises which they have not the least hope of fulfilling. In politics, people are still at an evolutionary stage where reasoning is dominated by the herd instinct, and so they are carried away by the candidate's oratory or personality or both.

The harmful effects of the activities of the individuals beset with serious and often abnormal psycho-physical defects are present in all areas of life. We have to face the fact that it is not the people who are out to do harm to their fellow-beings who are setting back the clock of civilization today, but, on the contrary, it is those misguided people who devote themselves to the uplifting of humankind, while remaining themselves under the influence of perverted emotions and prejudices. The history of our social plan of the last three hundred years is replete with attempts to reform on specific "end-gaining" principles, which even when achieved, lead to more complications, social conflict, and harmful diversity. If we are to stop this overbalancing, we must gradually raise the standard of individual psycho-physical co-ordination and pass to a stage of constructive, conscious control.

PART 4

SENSORY APPRECIATION IN ITS RELATION TO HAPPINESS

SENSORY APPRECIATION IN ITS RELATION TO HAPPINESS

The characteristic note of true happiness is struck when the healthy child is busily engaged in doing something which interests it. It is the natural desire of every child to find out "how it works." They are always attracted by machinery (in the broadest sense of the word). It is therefore very significant that in schools where experiments have been made in re-education on a general basis, the children have become more interested in this work than in any other of their school activities. They are not slow to recognize that they themselves are the most interesting machines, and their natural interest in mechanics finds full scope in their own re-education. This interest in the working of their own psycho-physical mechanisms grows steadily and comprehensively.

I can recall the expression of interest, happiness, and satisfaction shown by the child who understands for the first time that his or her unduly stiffened neck—with perhaps the head pulled too far back—is really not the neck's fault at all, but is caused by the fact of trying to do with the neck muscles what should be done by other parts of his or her mechanism.

(Note: Of course the teacher's manipulation will have given the child, previously, the reliable sensory appreciation in this connection.)

I cannot forget either the unfamiliar but satisfactory manifestations of the child who learns to inhibit—that is, to say "No" to some stimulus to misdirected activity—and then, with a confident expression, to give directions which are the result of a reasoned conception of the "means" of doing something. This whole process tends to prevent over-excitement of the fear reflexes.

(Note: With regard to changes in expression: One little girl who came for lessons had developed the most pronounced bad habits in the use of her organism and had what we call a "dour" expression when she first came. She became able to inhibit her reaction to   the stimulus which had previously started up the whole train of movements that were incorrect and harmful. When she first realized this, her whole demeanor changed. The fact that she could not only think out but control the means by which she could do something robbed her of the diffidence which had been such an overdeveloped characteristic in her case, and her former "dour" expression changed to one of confidence and happiness.)

I believe also that the majority of adults today lack real happiness because they are experiencing, not improvement, but continuous deterioration in their use of themselves. This is associated with those defects and unwanted traits of character, disposition, temperament, etc., which are characteristic of badly co-ordinated people struggling through life beset with maladjustments of the psycho-physical organism. All this sets up irritation and pressure during both sleeping and waking hours. As long as these maladjustments remain present, the malconditions increase day by day and week by week, and, not surprisingly, foster "unhappiness." Irritation is not compatible with happiness. Every effort made in daily life by the human being whose organism is already in such an irritated condition must tend to make that person even more so and diminish his or her chances of happiness as time goes on. Furthermore, happy experiences become of ever shorter duration until at last the person is forced into a state of unhappiness, a psycho-physical condition as disturbed as that state of ill-health which people reach when they experience a perverted form of satisfaction from pain—that is, in "the enjoyment of ill health," as we say.

People suffering irritation and pressure will be upset by experiences which would not have the least effect on someone whose sensory appreciation is reliable. Such people will also suffer comparative "failure" in their everyday activities and there can be nothing worse than "failure" in its effect on our emotions, self-respect, happiness, or confidence and on our temperament and character in general. Compare the general demeanor of someone who experiences success to one who fails. Success has a striking influence in this respect and is conducive to happiness, whether it be general success or success in making some simple movement. Confidence is born of success, not of failure. Our processes in education and in the general art of living must be based on principles which, through attention to the *means* an end may be secured, make certain of a large percentage of the satisfactory experiences which develop confidence, and reduce the number of unsatisfactory experiences which undermine our confidence and make us unhappy.

A medical specialist sent one of his patients to me for diagnosis. He asked me for my conclusions and when I said that his patient would be difficult to re-educate because of his unusually unbalanced emotional and irritable state, he told me: "He has been soured by failure in his professional work."

To further illustrate these points, we will consider the practical experiences of a person in recreation and sport, because we may assume that he or she participates in such activities in order to experience some happiness. We all know of the pleasurable anticipation and mild excitement of people who play golf, tennis, cricket, and other forms of recreation. Playing such games makes us happy, or should do. However, in the great majority of cases, this happiness tends to decrease the more we play: The reason for this will be clear if we think about the psycho-physical experiences in action and reaction which result from a recreation such as golf.

Watch an ordinary man at his first golf lesson. Firstly, his sensory appreciation is very probably unreliable and he lacks co-ordination and, secondly, he has never been re-educated on a general basis. Unfortunately, this applies equally to the teacher which means that, in both cases, their knowledge of the use of the mechanisms they are about to employ is derived from unsatisfactory and even harmful subconscious experiences. They have little conscious knowledge of the use of these mechanisms either in theory or in practice, and even that little will be on a specific basis. The true relation of "cause and effect" on a general basis will not be given due consideration; the majority of effects (symptoms of some "cause") that they chance to recognize will not be treated as effects, but as "causes," and will be dealt with on the "end-gaining" principle.

The pupil is asked, for instance, to "hold the club" in a certain way, or to "keep his eye on the ball," and various other things he should or should not do to control parts of his organism at a particular time. The poor pupil, however, is psycho-physically incapable of carrying out the specific instructions given to him to enable him to overcome his difficulties and strike the ball. In fact, his difficulties will increase. Many players fail to keep their eye on the ball, and, like the teachers, are unaware of the fundamental impeding psycho-physical factors involved in this failure.

It is not possible to discuss golf in detail in this book, but I will deal with the pupil's attempts to carry out the teacher's instructions from the standpoint of reliability of sensory appreciation and of co-ordination on a general basis. Firstly, no practical help is given to the pupil in this direction. The teacher cannot diagnose whether the pupil is co-ordinated generally or not. He simply assumes that if he gives the pupil certain instructions, he has conscientiously performed his task as a teacher. Yet, he should know that in swinging the club up and down, for instance, a number of different instructions must be performed by a number of different parts of the mechanism, and that these instructions must be linked together. The pupil, then, must be able to put more than one thing at a time into practice. However, the teacher cannot give the pupil any *means* of achieving this necessary co-ordination. The pupil's experiences, therefore, will inevitably be those which result from his efforts to learn in his ill-equipped condition.

After the first attempt at a stroke, some fault or faults will be pointed out by the teacher; the pupil will start to "concentrate" on the different corrections given and will *try* to make another stroke. He will already have decided that one or other of the corrections is the all-important one, and will concentrate specially on it to the virtual exclusion of all the others. This process is repeated with each attempt to strike the ball.

Although he may succeed in eradicating some specific faults in this way, he will do so by overlooking some other equally important corrections because he has concentrated on one at a time. This process of concentration adds to his list of difficulties (see earlier chapter). In addition, the process causes his fear reflexes to be over-excited and he gradually builds up an emotional state which impedes his progress at golf and becomes an established phobia influencing all his other activities. Thus, a state of comparative unhappiness is brought about.

One of the greatest factors in human development is the building up of confidence, which comes as a result of learning the correct *means* of gaining an end. By this method, relative success will come from the outset. Satisfactory psycho-physical experiences will follow, and with them that intelligent confidence and happiness which is the "consummated conquest" of the human being on a conscious plane.

In a civilization such as ours—where unrest, unhappiness, and lack of interest in the real things of life are strikingly manifest— all our efforts should be directed towards enabling the adult human being to retain the interest and satisfaction shown by the healthy child when using his or her organism successfully. We should create conditions in which satisfactory growth continues throughout life, and in which the stagnation which goes with fixed habits and specific "end-gaining" uses of the psycho-physical organism will be impossible.

Conscious use of the mechanism on a basis of general co-ordination in all the acts of living constitutes a real and never-ending intellectual problem of constructive control, which develops the interest and general intellectual pleasure in even such ordinary acts as "sitting down" and "standing up."

Take, for example, the act of "sitting down." The subconsciously controlled person, as soon he touches the chair, proceeds to "sit down"—that is, he "slumps" —*and as far as his awareness* is concerned the act of sitting is then completed. He remains oblivious to the misuse of the mechanisms involved and to the irritation and pressure associated with the harmful slump he has subconsciously assumed and which *feels* natural and comfortable. Likewise, with "standing up." Once he has stood up, the process is completed, again *as far as his awareness is concerned*. In both instances he ends a psycho-physical process which, in reality, *should never be finished*. His standard of awareness is as inadequate as his sensory appreciation is unreliable, and the psycho-physical conditions indicated here are inseparable from lack of interest and general pleasure in the ordinary acts of life. On the other hand, when a person sits down or stands up using constructive, conscious control, the process involves an adequate and continuous state of increasing awareness, growth, and development.

(Note: As I wrote in *Man's Supreme Inheritance*, "When real conscious control has been obtained, a 'habit' need never become fixed. It is not truly a habit at all, but a series of directions given to the subordinate controls of the body, which are carried out until countermanded.")

Conscious fundamental psycho-physical processes do not end. In all acts of life, the establishment of constructive control and continuous growth is inseparable from that manifestation we call "happiness." This comes from the application of the "means" and not the "end-gaining" principles which are adopted on a specific basis in the pursuit of "pleasure." Here we have the explanation of the growing need amongst subconsciously controlled people for *specific* pleasure, with all its attendant shortcomings of unrest and excess.

Unfortunately, we have been taught that all the ordinary acts of life should be automatic and unconscious. For this reason they have become indifferent. Such a psycho-physical condition induces stagnation in the organism. As it is a condition which becomes more and more pronounced with advancing age, we gradually lose the capacity to take conscious interest in and derive pleasure from those normal and useful activities of doing, hearing, seeing, etc. Small wonder, then, that sooner or later we seek satisfaction in less normal and less useful activities and create an undue demand for *specific* excitements and stimulations.

All our efforts in education should go into creating conditions in which growth will continue through life and where the stagnation which accompanies fixed habits will be impossible. We shall not then find men and women, as we do now, actually afraid to retire from their profession because they have no interest in doing anything else, and cannot adapt to a new way of life. This tragedy is one of the most common and poignant features of modern life: In such cases, the people concerned have so little control of their psycho-physical mechanisms (except within certain limited spheres) that they cannot use them in a new situation without experiencing the most distressing forms of psycho-physical functioning.

The processes of reasoning and action in the subconsciously controlled person about to retire from work reveal a tendency to fall back and depend more and more on automatic methods of procedure—repeating the same round of psycho-physical activities every day, and gradually limiting themselves further as time goes on. At the same time, the defects in the general use of the mechanism become more and more pronounced. Thus, with the approach of old age, stagnation and deterioration are gradually being cultivated throughout the organism: the very worst possible preparation for the new way of life ahead. This explains why so many people break down when they stop work.

(Note: Note the attitude of people in general towards circumstances, even in domestic life, which force changes in their habits of life. They have exaggerated, harmful conceptions of the discomfort and suffering they must endure because of this disturbance of the automatic round of their existence.)

Someone has said about the monotony of the environment in which we live, that monotony is the deathbed of existence. But what of the monotony *within* the self, a monotony caused by the gradual cessation of those sensations concerned with new experiences which have accompanied growth and mobility within the organism since birth? This is, indeed, monotony in its most harmful form, because it goes hand in hand with stagnation throughout the whole organism. We recognize, for instance, the danger of stagnation in our cells when they fail to repair wasted tissue. This stagnation is analogous to that which follows the cessation of sensations concerned with new experiences mentioned above, both forms of stagnation bringing monotony and unhappiness.

Yet another form of monotony results from "knowing," from having "grown up"; from the consciousness that we have ceased to grow. When a person concludes that he or she "knows" all there is to know about his subject, he decides, consciously or subconsciously, that there is nothing more to learn and promptly begins to lose what he does know. When he believes he has "grown up," he reaches a stage where he has begun to stultify those potentialities for growth which once were his, and monotony and discontent soon follow the establishment of this condition.

People who are satisfied that they "know" are the least observant people, and the least happy. Most people will admit that realization too often is not equal to anticipation, but again this is due to the psycho-physical conditions present. If realization is to equal or even sometimes to surpass anticipation, our psycho-physical plan of development must be fundamentally one of continuous growth and new experiences. We never reach the point when we finish learning. This gives us a continuous anticipation of new experiences. Realization of some new experience in psycho-physical functioning does not bring a sense of finality—with the consequent loss of interest—but is a clear indication that a step forward has been made in development, which is again a stepping stone to the next stage, and so on.

William James said we should get up every morning looking for health. I hope to go farther, because I offer a technique which will command for the human being an increasingly high standard of psycho-physical functioning which makes for health. The all-important duty of people in our present stage of evolutionary vicissitudes, is that of the *continuous* individual cultivation of fundamental, constructive conscious control of the psycho-physical organism and its potentialities.

It is true that humankind has made a specific application of so-called conscious control in the use of our reasoning powers in relation to "causes and effects," "means and consequences" outside of the human organism. But this attempt at specific control of environment has not resulted in a really reliable control of actual consequences. Our experiences seem to show that the more we apply this form of unreliable "conscious control," the worse off we are likely to be. I am convinced that if we are ever to command a reliable constructive control of environment and a satisfactory reasoning about "causes and effects," we must primarily be able to command fundamental constructive conscious control of the individual psycho-physical organism. To do this we need a higher and higher standard of psycho-physical functioning, which in turn demands a growing understanding and conscious use of the wonderful mechanisms concerned. Such a process provides the human creature with a sphere of psycho-physical activity which is almost unlimited in its possibilities.

Conclusions

Psycho-Physical Attitude

In this book, I have dealt with various human defects, peculiarities, shortcomings, and imperfections in the use of the psycho-physical organism, which tend to increase throughout life and too often become established as "bad habits" long before adolescence has been reached. The sum total of the experiences involved in this process is the foundation of what is called "mental attitude."

The attitude of the individual towards the functioning of the psycho-physical self, and to the use of his or her self in daily activities, is the "be all and end all." Only those who hold the key to this storehouse of their psycho-physical experiences, inherited or acquired, can reach that stage of understanding of their reactions to stimuli which justifies an optimistic view of any efforts to be made for humankind's uplifting.

The above-mentioned understanding is that of the psycho-physical processes, present at the various stages of the human being's growth and development, which are responsible for certain manifestations. A proper understanding of these manifestations is essential to any satisfactory consideration of "cause and effect," primarily in connection with the activities concerned with the development of the individual human beings themselves and, secondly, with their activities outside themselves in the complex round of civilized life. Humans continue to rush from one extreme to another on the "end-gaining" principle, in their efforts at reform or "physical" improvement. The point just made regarding an understanding of "cause and effect" is of the utmost importance in any estimate of schemes for the uplifting of humankind. What probability is there that any one of these schemes of reform will do anything but make conditions more chaotic, until the individuals concerned have been re-educated on a general basis and reorganized as a psycho-physical unity? For in the last analysis, it is the *individual's* reaction to the stimuli resulting from his or her *individual* conception of that scheme of reform that matters, even if the scheme, taken by itself, might be considered a satisfactory one.

This leads us back to the theme of conception which has been outlined. I have attempted to show that only in a state of *co-ordinated activity*, in which the organism is functioning near its maximum, can we hope for anything approaching a satisfactory conception of new and unfamiliar ideas or experiences. Hence the necessity of having an understanding of "cause and effect," primarily in connection with the functioning of the organism itself.

It is only after we have solved this problem in the individual that we can safely pass on to the secondary consideration of "cause and effect" in the problems of our daily life. Only then can we assert that individual reactions to stimuli will be those of a controlled human creature, whose employment of reasoning in life's activities prevents the undue and harmful excitement of the fear reflexes and emotions—especially when dealing with new and unfamiliar situations or problems which are the natural outcome of all processes tending towards advancement on the evolutionary plane.